D0982805

CRISIS:
Heterosexual Behavior in the Age of AIDS

WILLIAM H. MASTERS, M.D.
VIRGINIA E. JOHNSON
ROBERT C. KOLODNY, M.D.

GROVE PRESS
New York

Copyright © 1988 by William H. Masters, M.D., Virginia E. Johnson,
and Robert C. Kolodny, M.D.

Published by Grove Press, Inc.
920 Broadway
New York, N.Y. 10010

Library of Congress Cataloging-in-Publication Data

Masters, William H.
CRISIS : heterosexual behavior in the age of AIDS.

Bibliography: p.
Includes index.
1. AIDS (Disease)—Epidemiology.   2. AIDS (Disease)
—Prevention.   3. Safe sex in AIDS prevention.
I. Johnson, Virginia E.   II. Kolodny, Robert C.
III. Title.
RA644.A25M38   1988   616.9'79205   87-37175
ISBN 0-8021-1049-5

Designed by Irving Perkins Associates

Manufactured in the United States of America

First Edition 1988

10 9 8 7 6 5 4 3 2 1

CONTENTS

PREFACE

AIDS is a frightening disease. The fears engendered by the AIDS epidemic tap into the very roots of our human condition: fear of the unknown, fear of blood, fear of sex, fear of disease, fear of helplessness, fear of desertion and loneliness, fear of death. Such fears are not, of course, entirely irrational. AIDS is a killer, and our uncertainty about the exact magnitude of the AIDS epidemic only magnifies our anxieties.

There is also a darker underside to these anxieties. The fears provoked by the AIDS epidemic have led to acts of bigotry, discrimination, callousness, and even destructiveness. People infected with the AIDS virus have been stigmatized as though they chose to be infected. Entire groups of people—most notably, homosexual and bisexual men and intravenous drug users—have been vilified, cast as expendable commodities best left to the ravages of contagion. Judging from public reactions, many people seem to believe that these pariahs should be wiped from the face of the earth in apt retribution for their social and moral deviance. This is distressing, because it is only by recognizing the dignity of others that we can maintain our own human dignity, as the world learned from another holocaust at another time.

This book is not principally about AIDS as a disease. It is a research-based book that documents how extensively infection with the AIDS virus has spread beyond the original high-risk groups. In these pages, we explain in detail—and in very practical terms—why and how we as individuals and as a society must turn from a sense of relative complacency in dealing with the realities of the currently exploding epidemic and make a personal and public commitment to prevention as a primary issue. We also present some hard-hitting facts about real but generally ignored risks of infection with this insidious virus—risks that many scientists, public health experts, and researchers have generally been unwilling to acknowledge publicly, although in private they will often admit to concern about these very issues.

One thing is absolutely clear: until a cure is found, the best weapon we have in the fight against AIDS is information. But information that suggests scientific certainty where no such certainty exists, or information that presents an optimistic outlook primarily to prevent panic and hysteria, is a violation of the responsibility that scientists should vigorously protect and that the public should vociferously demand.

Some of what we have to say will be controversial. Some of our findings and recommendations will be belittled because they challenge the consensus that has been comfortably developed as one way of dealing with the raging epidemic of AIDS. But to ignore our findings, or to dismiss our cautionary interpretations of trends and problems in confronting this epidemic simply because they do not conform to the much-repeated official reassurances, is to approach a vast public health problem with clouded vision.

Several acknowledgments are in order for a project of this scope. The core research that provided the impetus for this book was conducted by Robert C. Kolodny, M.D., under the auspices of the Behavioral Medicine Institute. Nancy J. Kolodny, M.A., M.S.W., provided an extraordinary amount of assistance in collating the research data and carefully critiquing and editing all drafts of the book manuscript. Charles Rembar, a longtime friend, offered enthusiastic encouragement and meticulous, thoughtful advice in the early stages of the book project—in fact, without him, this book would not have come to fruition. Fred Jordan, our editor, had the vision to see the importance of the project from the very beginning and made many useful suggestions as the manuscript evolved. In every way, it has been a pleasure for us to work with Fred, whose publishing professionalism is of the highest order. Special mention should also be made of Joy Johannessen at Grove Press: her copy-editing skills are exemplary, and her accessibility was much appreciated.

Last, but certainly not least, we must voice our gratitude to the many people who participated in this research. They are, in the truest sense, our collaborators.

W. H. M.
V. E. J.
R. C. K.

1
BREAKING OUT

Hundreds of millions of words have been written about the global epidemic of AIDS—acquired immune deficiency syndrome. Regrettably, much of what has been written has simply been incorrect. In part, these inaccuracies are a result of the early clustering of cases in the United States and Europe among homosexual and bisexual men and intravenous drug abusers—groups that could be quickly and somewhat comfortably (at least in certain circles) categorized as "deviant," so that there was both an attitude of moral superiority toward and a sense of personal insulation from the epidemic. (As Stephen Jay Gould put it, "If AIDS had been first imported from Africa into a Park Avenue apartment, we would not have dithered as the exponential march began."[1]) In addition, misinformation about AIDS has resulted from a form of benevolent deception practiced by the scientific community: in the understandable wish to avoid mass panic, numerous pronouncements about AIDS were deliberately presented in the most optimistic light possible when even a healthy degree of scientific skepticism about the unknown would have produced a different, more realistic response. Compounding these sources of inaccuracies has been an alarming neglect of fundamental, systematic research into the mode of transmission of the AIDS virus—most notably, a surprising neglect of sound, sophisticated research into the specific associations of various forms of sexual behavior with the spread of this infection.

In later chapters we will point to many instances of misinformation that the general public has been fed about AIDS. First, however, we will introduce the alarming conclusion we have reached, based on our own research and studies conducted by others: contrary to claims by various government agencies and public health experts that infection with the AIDS virus is still largely confined to the original "high-risk" groups (gay and bisexual men and intravenous drug users), the epidemic has clearly broken out into the broader population and is continuing, even now, to make its silent inroads of infection while many maintain an attitude of complacency, not realizing that they too are at risk. We also conclude, categorically, that infection with the AIDS virus does *not* require intimate sexual contact or sharing of intravenous needles: transmission can, and does, occur as a result of person-to-person contact in which blood or other body fluids from a person who is harboring the virus are splashed onto or rubbed against someone else, even if this is a single, isolated occurrence.

At this point it is important to say that we do not make such assertions lightly, nor are we ignorant of their potential to provoke personal fear, social paranoia, and discriminatory behavior. Discrimination and paranoia are of course to be deplored; but in our judgment, realistic fear can both foster a better intellectual perspective on the issue of AIDS and be a powerful motivator of behavioral change—change, in this instance, being for many people a key to survival.

BREAKING OUT:
SOME BACKGROUND FACTS

The public has been generally lulled into believing that infection with the AIDS virus is still largely confined to homosexual and bisexual males and intravenous (IV) drug abusers,[2] but this view of the underside of the AIDS epidemic is extraordinarily erroneous. Here are the fundamental facts behind such a statement.

Authorities are greatly underestimating the number of people infected with the AIDS virus in the population today. No epidemic of sexually transmitted disease has ever stood still, numerically speaking, without the availability of a preventive vaccine or a cure. Yet most medical experts continue to claim that there are only 1.5 million people infected with the AIDS virus today, which is the same estimate that was made in mid-1986 by the U.S. Public Health Service in collaboration with the Centers for Disease Control (CDC).[3] Even if the AIDS virus is far less contagious than other sexually transmitted viruses (e.g., herpes, hepatitis B), the fact is that most people harboring the AIDS virus—and unknowingly transmitting it to others—don't realize they're infected. Many if not most of them are not taking any precautions in terms of sexual behavior, donating blood, or using IV drugs, so that they continue to infect others over an indefinite period of time. For this reason, it is quite likely that there are now 3 million or more "carriers" of the AIDS virus in the United States, most of whom are otherwise healthy and unaware of their infected, contagious state.[4] Although the situation in Europe, Canada, and Australia is not quite so far along—in general, the spread of the epidemic in these countries seems to be lagging two to three years behind that in the U.S.—in central Africa and Haiti AIDS is already decimating the populace.

Experts generally are gravely underestimating the degree to which the AIDS virus has spread into the heterosexual community. There have been several different mechanisms by which the AIDS virus "crossed over" from the original high-risk groups to the general population. Certainly, bisexual males represented one of the earliest vectors of this crossover. Probably more important, from a numerical viewpoint, was the pattern involving IV drug users. Here the fact that many female addicts work as prostitutes in order to support their drug habits was and continues to be of considerable importance. Since prostitutes have frequent sexual contact with numerous partners, and since many prostitutes do not insist that their customers use condoms, it is not hard to see how even a relatively small number of AIDS-infected prostitutes could infect large numbers of men. These men, not realizing that they were infected, could then transmit the AIDS virus to other female sex partners. Since this situation has now been festering over a period of more than five years, it can safely be estimated that the number of non-drug-using heterosexuals who have been infected in this manner by a sexual partner is substantial: probably on the order of 200,000 or more.

This is not the end of the story, however. Indications are that the AIDS virus is slowly but surely working its way into the younger population—the 15- to 24-year-old age group—which has, at least in the last quarter-century, been the primary wedge driving epidemics of sexually transmitted diseases (STDs) in the United States and elsewhere across the world.[5] (Admittedly, the identification of teenagers and very young adults who are infected with the AIDS virus has been ignored up until now, incomprehensibly, so this may still be a matter of some conjecture.)

Equally alarming is the not unexpected concentration of infection among heterosexuals with what used to be called "highly promiscuous" patterns of sexual behavior but might now be better labeled "sex with multiple partners." As the U.S. Surgeon General put it in his 1986 report, "The risk of infection increases according to the number of partners one has, *male or female*. The more partners you have, the greater the risk of becoming infected with the AIDS virus."[6] We will discuss this issue later in some detail; suffice it to say here that it is noteworthy for several distinct reasons.

First, people who elect to have numerous sexual contacts with multiple partners in the era of huge media campaigns about genital herpes and AIDS tend to be people who don't think they are personally at risk for these infections. (One bit of supportive evidence for this point: a CDC report of AIDS virus infection in two women involved in "social/sexual clubs" noted that of the 55 club members who were interviewed and asked if they "perceived themselves as being at risk of having AIDS," 40—73%—said they did not![7]) Their denial of risk not only allows them to maintain their pattern of sexual behavior in a relatively worry-free state but also means that they will be unlikely to use standard precautions for so-called safe sex, such as condoms or avoiding anal intercourse. Second, since these people are having sex with numerous partners, they are increasing the likelihood of spreading their infection, and the people *they* are infecting are in turn likely to expose large numbers of partners. This phenomenon is well known to workers in the field of sexually transmitted diseases; it can be said, in fact, that the most promiscuous 5% of those with a particular STD (such as syphilis or gonorrhea) serve as a conduit for more than half of the overall cases of that illness in any region. Third, people who are engaging in sex with large numbers of partners are also likely to be participating in a greater variety of sex acts than their more staid counterparts.[8] This means that they are more likely than other, less sexually adventuresome people to have oral-genital contact or anal intercourse—which may increase the probability of spreading the infection.

The breakout of AIDS into the heterosexual community in the United States should come as no particular surprise. In Africa, for example, reported cases of AIDS are about equally divided between men and women, and relatively few cases can be traced to homosexual or bisexual contact.[9] Similarly, in Haiti the percentage of AIDS cases found in women has been steadily rising: from 14% in 1980–82 to 36% in 1985[10] to almost 50% today.[11] It is likely that heterosexual transmission of AIDS will soon become the predominant mechanism of infection on a worldwide basis.

The more people who are infected with the AIDS virus, the more quickly the rate of spread escalates (until behavior patterns change in a meaningful way). Two experts at the CDC expressed it this way:

> As the prevalence of infection in the population increases, the likelihood of infection in a random partner also increases. Therefore, in an epidemic, one would expect to observe an increasing risk of infection as the prevalence of the infection increases.[12]

All these considerations point in one direction: AIDS is breaking out. The AIDS virus is now running rampant in the heterosexual community. Unless something is done to contain this global epidemic, we face a mounting death toll in the years ahead that will be the most formidable the world has ever seen.

SOME NEW FINDINGS ON AIDS VIRUS INFECTION IN HETEROSEXUALS

Because we began to worry in late 1985 that AIDS was breaking out of the original high-risk groups, we tried to devise a strategy for assessing the prevalence of infection with the AIDS virus in the heterosexual population. Following Sutton's Law,* we decided that the best opportunity for identifying a new trend in its earliest stages

---

*Reportedly, the famous bank robber Willie Sutton, when asked why he robbed banks, concisely noted, "That's where the money is." In medicine, Sutton's Law means using the diagnostic test or investigative method most likely to reveal the solution.

7

would be among heterosexuals who had a large number of sex partners each year. To avoid the hornet's nest of complications that would arise in a study of prostitutes (for example, that their widespread use of intravenous drugs could cloud the mode of transmission of the virus), we chose a different approach. We set out to examine a geographically and socially diverse group of non-monogamous heterosexual men and women, along with a comparison group of heterosexual men and women in long-term monogamous relationships.

To do this, we obtained a sample of 800 sexually active heterosexual adults between the ages of 21 and 40 who all met three criteria:

1. No blood transfusions received from 1977 on
2. No use of illicit drugs by injection
3. No homosexual or bisexual contact from 1977 on

These 800 adults consisted of the following groups: 200 men and 200 women who reported having been in long-term monogamous relationships (either marriage or co-habitation) for at least five years prior to the time of being interviewed; 200 men and 200 women who reported a minimum of 6 sexual partners a year over the preceding five years (regardless of whether they were married). Study participants in both groups were drawn from major metropolitan areas in four different geographic regions, the Northeast, the South, the Midwest, and the West.

All study subjects completed a self-administered questionnaire and were interviewed to obtain a detailed sex history covering the preceding five years, as well as information regarding prior sexually transmitted diseases, past and current contraceptive practices, and each subject's personal sense of being at risk for genital herpes and AIDS. A blood sample taken from each subject was tested for antibody to the AIDS virus.

Summarizing the results here (for a more detailed discussion of this research, see Chapter 4), we should note the following points:

- The average annual number of sex partners in the nonmonogamous group was 11.5 for the women, 9.8 for the men. In contrast (and by definition), the average annual number of sex partners in the monogamous group was 1.

- The prevalence of infection with the AIDS virus among the 400 strictly monogamous men and women was, not surprisingly, very low: only 1 out of the 400, or 0.25%, had evidence of such an infection.

- In contrast, the prevalence of infection with the AIDS virus among the 400 men and women with numerous sexual partners was strikingly higher: 14 women (7%) and 10 men (5%).

- Among the subgroup of nonmonogamous persons who averaged more than 12 sex partners annually, the prevalence of infection with the AIDS virus was even higher: 14% for women, 12% for men.

- Nonmonogamous subjects were more likely than monogamous subjects to have engaged in anal intercourse over the preceding five years; furthermore, for those subjects in either sample who did engage in anal intercourse, the frequency of this type of sexual contact was approximately three

9

times higher in the nonmonogamous group than in the monogamous group.

- Relatively few of the men and women who had numerous sex partners each year considered themselves at risk for contracting the AIDS virus. Almost none of the women in this group routinely asked their sex partners to use condoms; none of the males had used condoms routinely and consistently in the twelve months preceding the time of their interviews.

The implications of this research are relatively straightforward. If there is a significant rate of infection with the AIDS virus among heterosexuals who are very active with a number of different sex partners, it follows that much larger numbers of people are being exposed. In the case of our study, for example, if each of the 24 infected people in the nonmonogamous group is having sex with 15 others in the course of a year, then these 24 people have directly exposed 360 people to the virus through their sexual meanderings. If each of these 360 people has sexual contact with 5 additional partners, an additional 1,800 persons will have been potentially exposed by the original group of 24. In contrast, the one person who tested positive in the monogamous group is probably exposing only his spouse—or possibly caught this infection *from* his spouse (who did not participate in the study).

As larger numbers of people are exposed, larger numbers of infections are transmitted, both sexually and otherwise. With time—perhaps within just a few years—there will be a "trickle-down effect" in which infection with the AIDS virus will be commonplace, not just in persons who have had many sex partners, but in heterosexuals who have had relatively few sex partners in their lives. While the infection spreads, it will be possible to maintain a certain degree of blind complacency by simply counting and classifying actual cases of AIDS. This will comfort those who use the absence of a great leap in the percentage of AIDS cases occurring among non-drug-using heterosexuals as "proof" that the virus is still contained largely in the homosexual/bisexual/ drug-using communities. But with a disease that often has a latency period of five years or more from the time of initial infection until the diagnosis can be definitively established,[13] we are ignoring biological reality if we accept such proof.

We are not talking about a disease that is simply an embarrassment or an inconvenience: AIDS, so far as we now know, is a disease that is invariably fatal. And though it has not been determined how many of those infected with the AIDS virus will eventually come down with AIDS, it looks right now as though the percentage will be quite high. Thus, the implications of the spread of the AIDS virus into the general population are frightening. As others have said, the AIDS epidemic carries the potential to be the greatest natural tragedy in human history.

THE NUMBERS OF A GLOBAL EPIDEMIC

In 1986 a spokesman for the World Health Organization estimated that on a global basis there were 100,000 cases

11

of AIDS, 300,000 to 500,000 people with other symptoms of infection with the AIDS virus, and somewhere between 5 million and 10 million symptom-free carriers of the virus, many of whom will ultimately develop full-blown cases of AIDS.[14] By late 1987 45,000 cases of AIDS had been reported in the United States alone. In Western Europe about 7,000 cases had been reported. In Africa about 50,000 cases had probably occurred. Indeed, cases had been identified in more than 110 countries, including Russia, Japan, Australia, India, and the People's Republic of China.

These numbers are, we believe, serious underestimates of the actual number of cases that have occurred. There are several explanations for such underreporting. In some countries, for instance, there were clearly political overtones to the issue, especially in the early days of the epidemic. To report an alarmingly large number of cases of AIDS was to run the risk of decreased tourism, with its economic consequences, and to admit to a major public health problem, which might be taken by some to imply unhygienic conditions, inadequate public education, and so forth. Furthermore, many countries were unwilling, because of their religious or cultural heritage, to acknowledge a problem that initially seemed to be concentrated among homosexuals, bisexuals, and IV drug abusers.

In the United States and Europe there were several different problems that together resulted in substantial underreporting, which to a large degree has continued up until the present. First, physicians in many locales could not diagnose AIDS because they were not personally familiar with the syndrome. (Most physicians who graduated from medical school before 1979 probably never encountered a case in school or in their postgraduate training.) Second, until the blood test for antibody to the AIDS virus became available in mid-1985, the diagnosis was chiefly made on the basis of clinical recognition, with little direct laboratory evidence to support a physician's impression. Third, some physicians have used other diagnoses, euphemistic or misleading, in order to protect patients and their families from the ignominy of a diagnosis of AIDS. (Recall, for example, the situation with regard to Liberace and Roy Cohn.) We estimate that for this reason alone, 20% of all AIDS cases in the United States and Europe have not been reported.[15]

In a variation on this theme, many physicians do not report cases of AIDS until after the patient has died. This may sometimes be because the physician fears that becoming known as an "AIDS doctor" will adversely affect his or her practice. It may also reflect other considerations. For instance, a physician may be motivated by a strongly humanitarian urge in such situations. Sometimes the motivation is more questionable, though, as in the case of Stewart McKinney, a congressman from Connecticut, whose illness with AIDS appears to have been concealed from the electorate despite rumors of his condition; while his death from AIDS was finally acknowledged, such instances of delayed reporting, if common, would badly skew the government's efforts to monitor the rate of increase of the disease and its geographic distribution.

The other major reason for a significant underestimate of the actual number of AIDS cases was a technical one: between 1982 and late 1987 the CDC insisted on unduly restrictive criteria for diagnosing cases of AIDS,[16] as many workers in the field pointed out. Although there was certainly some scientific rationale for maintaining a relatively unchanging set of diagnostic criteria (as the CDC itself noted, such a case definition "has provided useful data on disease trends because it is precise, consistently interpreted, and highly specific"[17]), there were marked disadvantages too. Once it became clear in 1985 that emaciation and dementia were common features of the AIDS syndrome, and that thousands of infected people who were showing these symptoms were in fact severely ill (with many going on to die), it was a curious form of scientific denial not to permit these cases to be diagnosed as AIDS. The result of this insistence on unrealistically narrow criteria for case reporting was not just to underestimate the number of cases but to make it seem that the rate of increase in the overall number of AIDS cases in the U.S. was declining, when in fact just the opposite was happening.

The bottom line of all of these considerations is that there has been such serious underreporting of the actual incidence of AIDS that the statistics as of late 1987 were off by some 50%. This means that in the U.S. there has probably been a cumulative total of at least 67,000 cases of AIDS from the time the epidemic began until the end of 1987. In Africa, where underreporting is even more serious, it is likely that the cumulative total as of the end of 1987 was 100,000 or more.

This problem is not just an academic one. If the baseline number of cases used by epidemiologists and public health officials to estimate future trends of this epidemic has been off by so much to begin with, then "official" estimates of the toll the world will see in the future are also far too conservative. For example, the U.S. Public Health Service has estimated that by the end of 1991 there will be a cumulative total of 270,000 cases of AIDS in this country alone, with 179,000 deaths.[18] But this estimate was based on the "official" reported statistics available as of mid-1986. Today, taking into account the strong probability of a larger baseline number of cases even at that time,[19] as well as more realistic estimates of the rate of conversion from the symptomless stage of infection with the AIDS virus to the full-blown AIDS syndrome, we believe that by the end of 1991 the actual number of AIDS cases in America will exceed 500,000, with more than 300,000 deaths. Worldwide there will be at least 2 million cases of AIDS, with well over 1 million deaths. By the year 2000, unless astonishing progress is made in the development of a vaccine to prevent this infection, there will be a cumulative total of 5 million cases of AIDS in America alone. Worldwide there will be 25 million cases. The enormity of this threat—and the world's failure to respond swiftly enough with both funding for research and planning for this frightening future—should not be taken lightly.

2

AIDS: THE VIRUS
AND ITS TRANSMISSION

How the AIDS epidemic originated is a matter of much conjecture. In retrospect, it appears that there was a case of infection with the AIDS virus in a teenage boy in St. Louis in 1969.[1] This raises the possibility that the AIDS virus may have appeared sporadically in the United States several times before it ignited an epidemic. Before this case became known, the most plausible explanation for how the AIDS epidemic began drew on the close similarity, both in structure and in certain types of immunologic effects, between the AIDS virus and a virus that affects monkeys, causing a type of illness that closely resembles AIDS.[2] It is possible either that this virus mutated into a form affecting humans or that the initial cases of AIDS in Africa actually represented human infections by a simian virus.

Because of their rarity, and because no such disease officially existed at the time, the earliest cases of unusual infections and rare cancers resulting from suppression of the immune system by the AIDS virus were not identified as AIDS and were only reported after the initial cluster of cases in the United States was finally recognized as a "new" illness in 1981.[3] Several retrospective studies, using African blood samples obtained in the early and mid-1970s for other purposes but frozen and stored since then, have shown that antibodies to the AIDS virus were present in humans as early as 1977.[4] Such documentation makes it difficult to believe that the AIDS virus originated in a top-secret government biological warfare project that somehow ran amok, as the Russian press has claimed.[5] And unless one believes that God had a particular gripe with the peoples of central Africa, it is hard to look at AIDS as a form of divine retribution with a moralistic twist.

THE AIDS VIRUS

AIDS is a deadly syndrome, or collection of clinical features, that is known to be caused by the human immunodeficiency virus (HIV, previously called HTLV-III or LAV). HIV damages the immune system—the system that ordinarily protects the body against infection—leaving a person especially susceptible to other infections and to a variety of malignancies. AIDS itself is actually the end stage of infection with HIV. In earlier stages of the infection, many people have no visible symptoms, whereas others experience various types of mild illness or more serious health problems that can be debilitating but do not fit the diagnostic criteria for a full-blown case of AIDS. (A discussion of the medical features of AIDS can be found in Appendix A.) While there is some uncertainty about how many of those infected with HIV will ultimately develop AIDS, it is increasingly apparent that the majority will eventually die of this disorder.[6]

In most cases, the AIDS virus is spread from one person to another either by sexual contact or by sharing intravenous drug needles and syringes. (Other, less common forms of transmission will be discussed later in this chapter.) Once inside the body, the virus vigorously attacks certain lymphocytes (a type of white blood cell), called T-helper cells, that ordinarily are the key coordinators of the immune system. The invasion is an intriguing one that is almost like a military operation. First, the AIDS virus seeks out and identifies the T-helper cells as targets. Next, it attaches itself to the outside of the cell, from which it will launch its actual attack. After penetrating the cell membrane, the virus sheds its outer protein coat, releasing a strand of genetic material called RNA (ribonucleic acid), which is transformed by a unique enzyme into several strands of DNA (deoxyribonucleic acid), another form of genetic material that carries important molecular coding for the production of amino acids and proteins within the cell. This DNA, acting something like a missile, then penetrates the nucleus of the T-helper cell, which is the heart of the cell's usual operations.

In the cell nucleus the DNA from the virus is combined with the host cell's own genetic code so that the host cell becomes, in effect, a mini-factory for producing copies of the virus. Every time the infected host cell divides, copies of the AIDS virus are produced along with more host cells, each of which contains the viral DNA code. Because the AIDS virus copying cycle is generally restricted until such time as the infected host cell is activated,[7] the entire process can be compared to planting tens of thousands of time bombs in a territory that is being invaded in preparation for later destruction. While the activation process is not fully understood at present, it seems that other infections (including hepatitis B, herpes, and possibly syphilis) may trigger such an event, raising the possibility that other infections may trigger multiplication of previously dormant HIV infection.[8] Once the T-helper cell is activated and the AIDS virus reproduces, the cell is killed. As a result, people with AIDS often have a low lymphocyte count. In fact, many people with HIV infection have a lowered lymphocyte count prior to getting AIDS. The drop in the number of lymphocytes may be a precursor of imminent malfunction in the immune system, since unusual infections that are often associated with AIDS are more likely to occur once the number of T-helper cells is depleted so much that the surviving cells cannot coordinate operations of the immune system very effectively.

The AIDS virus also selectively infects several other cells that are part of the immune system: B cells, monocytes, and macrophages. While these cells are not typically killed by HIV, even when it reproduces, their functioning as an integral part of the immune system is clearly disrupted. It is also thought that these cells may serve as an important reservoir for persistent viral infection in persons infected with HIV.[9]

In addition, the AIDS virus selectively attacks, invades, and destroys cells in the brain. Though the exact mechanism of this attack is not certain at present, one line of reasoning suggests that HIV infects monocytes outside the central nervous system. The infected monocytes then serve as a sort of Trojan horse for carrying the infection past the body's usually formidable line of defense for the brain itself, a protective filter known as the blood-brain barrier. Once inside the brain, the infected monocytes may release chemical substances that are toxic to brain cells, resulting in the various brain disorders frequently encountered in people with AIDS.

Despite uncertainties about some of the precise mechanisms involved in the biology of HIV infection, it is clear that this is a persistent infection. Because the AIDS virus's genetic coding is integrated into that of the host cells it attacks, "individuals who have been infected with HIV are permanently infected."[10]

TRANSMISSION

In the early 1980s there was considerable uncertainty about how AIDS was transmitted. Today, although medical authorities disagree on certain aspects of transmission, there is reasonable unanimity on a number of key points. These can be summarized as follows:

1. The AIDS virus is primarily spread by sexual contact.
2. Transfusions of infected blood or blood products also spread the AIDS virus.
3. Sharing or reusing of contaminated needles or syringes by IV drug abusers is another significant vector of transmission of the AIDS virus.

4. The AIDS virus is readily transmitted from mother to child during pregnancy and childbirth and may also be transmitted during breast-feeding.

5. Skin or mucous membrane contact with infected blood (and possibly other biological fluids) also transmits the AIDS virus.

Since understanding the various modes of transmission of the AIDS virus is central to understanding the risks of infection in different circumstances and the steps that must be taken for purposes of prevention, we will discuss each of these mechanisms in some detail.

SEXUAL TRANSMISSION

While there is general agreement that any sexual contact involving the exchange of biological fluids from one partner to another results in a risk of HIV transmission (if one partner is infected), there is a great deal of uncertainty about the exact magnitude of risk attending various types of sexual activity. The greatest risk seems to be associated with anal intercourse, in both homosexuals and heterosexuals.[11] This is partly because the tissue lining the rectum is relatively delicate and susceptible to tears,[12] but it may also reflect other factors, including a difference in the pH of the rectum compared to that of the vagina, a different microbial environment, or a difference in tissue resistance to penetration by the invading virus particles.

Vaginal intercourse is also conclusively known to transmit the AIDS virus, both from man to woman and from woman to man.[13] At present it appears that the risk

21

of infection from vaginal intercourse is considerably lower than the risk associated with anal intercourse, but this assessment is more guesswork than scientific certainty. In several studies of transmission of the AIDS virus from one spouse to the other, there has been no strong correlation with anal sex, suggesting that unprotected vaginal intercourse is also a frequent means of spreading the infection.[14] On the other hand, it has been estimated that the risk of an infected man's transmitting HIV to a woman through a single act of unprotected vaginal intercourse is approximately 1 in 1,000, while the risk of an infected woman's transmitting HIV to a man in a single act of unprotected vaginal intercourse is about 1 in 2,000.[15] We believe that these estimates are unduly optimistic, since we have preliminary evidence from our own research that the risk is about 1 in 400 for women and 1 in 600 for men.[16]

It has been clearly shown that the AIDS virus is present in relatively high concentrations in the semen of infected men.[17] It has also been shown that the AIDS virus is present in cervical and vaginal secretions,[18] although the concentrations of the virus seem to be somewhat lower in these fluids than in semen.[19] There doesn't seem to be any time during the menstrual cycle when the virus typically disappears, so from the viewpoint of potential infectivity, there is no such thing as a "safe" time in the woman's menstrual calendar. Because the menstrual flow carries the additional risk of blood mixing with cervical and vaginal secretions, there is a distinct possibility, as yet unconfirmed, that vaginal intercourse (or cunnilingus) during this time is more dangerous from the viewpoint of infectivity than when menstruation is not occurring.

There is much less certainty about whether HIV is spread by oral sex. The *Surgeon General's Report on Acquired Immune Deficiency Syndrome,* prepared in 1986, makes no mention of oral-genital transmission except for the following statement: "If you or your partner is at high risk, avoid mouth contact with the penis, vagina, or rectum."[20] Various studies have found no evidence of an increased risk of HIV infection linked to oral sex. For instance, Winkelstein and his co-workers,[21] reporting on a large prospective study of men in San Francisco (where they saw no evidence of HIV infection in heterosexual men), found that engaging in oral sex did not increase the risk of HIV infection among homosexual or bisexual men who had not engaged in anal sex.* Similarly, a study by Padian and her co-workers of 97 female sexual partners of men with HIV infection found no indication of a heightened risk of viral transmission associated with oral sex, although women who engaged in anal sex in addition to vaginal or oral sex were 2.3 times more likely to acquire HIV infection than those who did not.[22] However, none of the women in this study participated exclusively in oral sex, so it is quite possible that fellatio with

*Unfortunately, because they quantified oral sex only in terms of "none" or "some" rather than doing a more detailed frequency analysis, their results may have masked a significant influence of oral sex. That is, it might have been revealing to look at the subgroup of men who engaged in oral sex with a relatively high frequency (e.g., 100 times per year or more) compared to those who never engaged in oral sex or those who engaged in oral sex infrequently (e.g., fewer than 12 times a year).

23

ejaculation may *transmit* HIV even though it doesn't *increase* the risk of transmission above the level found with vaginal intercourse.

Despite these failures to find evidence suggesting that the AIDS virus can be transmitted by oral sex, other reports provide a different perspective. Possibly the most compelling is a 1987 study by Fischl and co-workers[23] that found strong statistical support for a link between oral sex and transmission of the AIDS virus in a study of 45 AIDS patients and their spouses, both male and female (26 of the 45 spouses, or 58%, showed evidence of HIV infection, indicating a high rate of sexual transmission among heterosexuals).* We have also seen two cases of HIV infection in exclusively homosexual males (ages 21 and 33) who had never engaged in anal sex but participated in oral-genital sex with high degrees of frequency.

Though there is as yet no research conclusively proving that the AIDS virus can be transmitted by oral sex, we want to stress that it is a virtual certainty that this mode of spreading the infection is real. For one thing, there is no known viral or bacterial STD that is *not* spread, at least at times, by oral-genital contact.[24] Furthermore, the difficulty of "proving" that oral-genital sex transmits the AIDS virus is largely an artifact: because it would be patently unethical to perform experiments on humans to try to prove the existence of this mode of transmission, we are forced to rely on somewhat

---

*Fischl and co-workers did, in fact, quantify the frequency of oral sex in their subjects, which may have allowed them to reach a more accurate conclusion. They defined "repeated oral sex" as "at least two contacts per month or 50% or more of total sexual activity."

oblique research strategies in which the actual effects of oral sex are generally masked due to other (confounding) sexual practices. Finally, it is perhaps even more likely that the mucous membrane lining of the mouth will have minor cuts, scratches, blisters, or abrasions both from eating and from using a toothbrush or dental floss than it is that the mucosa of the rectum will be torn during anal sex; that such lesions would provide an easy portal of entry for the virus—carried in either semen or vaginal secretions—is essentially unarguable.

There is even more skepticism about the AIDS virus being transmitted by kissing. Here again, there is no question that this route of transmission is possible. The AIDS virus has been isolated repeatedly from saliva;[25] other sexually transmitted diseases, including genital herpes and syphilis, can be spread in this manner; and the point just raised about the common existence of cuts, scratches, or abrasions on the lips or in the mouth is applicable, particularly in terms of "soul kissing" or "French kissing"—that is, deep, tongue-probing, saliva-mixing kisses.

Those who prefer to believe that the virus can't be spread by kissing cite two facts to make their case. The first is that the virus is present in lower concentrations in saliva than in semen or blood, which certainly appears to be true based on the relatively crude studies that have been done to date. However, there is probably enough live virus present to infect another person. The second fact, which is also true in a limited sense but of dubious comfort, is that so far no one has identified a case of AIDS in which kissing was the definite means of transmission. Yet this is just another instance in which the inability to experiment in a carefully controlled way creates confusion. Despite the importance of knowing whether kissing can actually transmit the AIDS virus, it is clearly unethical to conduct such studies with humans, and it is nonsensical to require such "proof" from real-life circumstances that are unlikely to arise very frequently within view of researchers.

It seems strange to have to raise such an obvious point, but if there are lingering uncertainties about the transmission of a deadly infection, shouldn't we be adopting precautions against the worst-case possibility rather than making the most optimistic assumption? After all, this is quite literally a life-and-death matter, not an intellectual discussion with purely philosophical ramifications. And yet the medical/scientific community has given the public a rather reassuring assessment suggesting that kissing is not apt to be a means of spreading the AIDS virus.[26] This raises the question of whether the intention behind such a posture is to inform people of the relevant risks or to take the path of least resistance, stressing only the proven dangers and virtually ignoring those that are possible but not yet thoroughly documented.

NONSEXUAL TRANSMISSION

The primary nonsexual mechanism of transmission of the AIDS virus is the use of needles or syringes contaminated with the blood of an already infected person. As a practical matter, this generally occurs when IV drug abusers share their "works," but it can also occur with other forms of needle sharing, as with intramuscular injections (sometimes athletes injecting drugs such as anabolic steroids share needles) or subcutaneous injections (known among drug users as "skin popping"). Although it is widely recognized that sharing contaminated needles will spread the AIDS virus, the risks of sharing syringes are less well known. A syringe can become contaminated when the drug user draws back on the plunger to see whether the needle is positioned in a vein, just as a doctor or nurse would do; if blood is easily drawn into the syringe, a vein has been tapped. The relatively small amount of blood in the syringe is quite enough to contain huge numbers of the AIDS virus, so that even when the original contents of the syringe are shot up and the residue of blood clinging to the walls of the syringe (and trapped at its mouth) is diluted with the volume of new drug to be injected, there is a high probability of transmitting the infection. One of the reasons for this, of course, is that the live virus is being pumped directly into the bloodstream, bypassing some of the body's ordinary defenses against infection, such as the skin.

One might think that given the avalanche of publicity about the danger of becoming infected with the AIDS virus by using contaminated needles or syringes, drug users would be much more cautious and the frequency of this means of transmission would show a significant drop. This has not occurred so far for two reasons. First, very few IV drug abusers exercise much caution, which shouldn't be surprising. They are trapped by an addictive impulse so strong, so compelling, that they regularly risk death by overdose or by the use of impure junk of uncertain chemical composition. The urgency of getting a "fix" when the body's appetite for a narcotic is scream-

27

ing obliterates virtually every other concern: shooting up as soon as the junk is available is an almost mandatory act under these circumstances, even if the needle is known to have been dipped in cyanide. Second, as the prevalence of HIV infection among drug addicts has risen over the last five years,[27] the likelihood of sharing a contaminated needle or syringe has risen dramatically. The mathematics behind this are fairly straightforward. If there is only a 10% prevalence of infection among drug addicts in a particular city, there is only a 1 in 10 chance that you will be infected with the virus if you share another addict's needle. If the prevalence of infection is 70% to 80%, the chances of infection are considerably higher and become a virtual certainty if you share unsterilized needles on a frequent basis. In addition, the greater the prevalence, the more the odds favor an addict's becoming infected earlier in his or her drug-using career.

The other major means of nonsexual transmission of the AIDS virus so far has been the transfusion of contaminated blood products, including not only "regular" blood transfusions (e.g., whole blood or blood components such as packed red blood cells or platelets) but also clotting factors that most hemophiliacs require to keep from bleeding uncontrollably. Of the estimated 20,000 people with hemophilia in the United States, about half of whom require weekly infusions of clotting factors, close to 75% are now infected with the AIDS virus, and most of them were infected prior to 1985.[28] While only a small percentage of infected hemophiliacs have gone on to develop full-blown cases of AIDS (which may just reflect the long latency time before the infection causes visible symptoms or illness), many authorities believe that most if not all of them will eventually come down with the disorder. There is some basis for hoping that the rate of HIV infection in hemophiliacs may decline in the future, since it has been found that heating the clotting factors generally appears to kill the AIDS virus.[29]

The risk of HIV infection among nonhemophiliacs receiving blood transfusions has been the subject of some controversy. Various experts from the government and the blood banking industry claim that no more than 4,000 cases of transfusion-transmitted AIDS theoretically occurred prior to the advent of blood testing in 1985.[30] Furthermore, only about 15% of this number had actually been diagnosed by the end of 1986.[31] Nevertheless, it is clear that 2% of AIDS cases in adults and almost 10% of the cases in children were a result of blood transfusions,[32] which also seemed to be the primary risk factor in 10% of the cases in women.[33]

Most experts claim that with better donor screening (to attempt to eliminate homosexual and bisexual men and IV drug abusers from the donor pool) and the availability of a highly sensitive test to detect antibody to the AIDS virus (allowing donated blood to be discarded if found to be infected), the nation's blood supply is now essentially safe from the threat of AIDS. We disagree with this contention and will present a detailed discussion of our reasoning in Chapter 5. Here we will simply point out that neither the donor exclusion criteria nor the screening antibody tests are foolproof, and it is a certainty that contaminated units of blood continue to slip through for use in transfusions.

One of the saddest aspects of the AIDS epidemic is

that the deadly virus is commonly transmitted from mother to child during pregnancy and childbirth. Experts estimate that 50% to 60% of infants born to infected women will be infected,[34] which is a particularly alarming statistic since HIV infection among women occurs principally in the childbearing years. HIV has also been identified in the breast milk of infected women,[35] and there is evidence that it can be transmitted postnatally: for example, in one case a woman who was infected by a postnatal blood transfusion passed the infection to her breast-feeding baby.[36]

There has been much discussion in recent years about whether the AIDS virus can be transmitted by nonsexual contact other than the mechanisms mentioned above. The discussion has largely focused on transmission by so-called casual contact, which has never been defined as specifically as one might wish. The general message has been that the AIDS virus is virtually never transmitted in this manner—and one of the arguments used to buttress this anxiety-reducing message has been that among the thousands of health care workers who have accidentally stuck themselves with needles used to draw blood from AIDS patients (or others known to be infected with HIV), there have been only a few instances of documented infection.[37]

This line of reasoning must be carefully reassessed in light of scientific common sense, dramatized by new data from the CDC. We have claimed for several years that as with other viral infections, anyone who is exposed to the blood or other infected body fluids of an HIV-infected person may in turn develop an HIV infection. This can occur, we said, because the skin is not always a perfect protective barrier to infection. If a person has a cut (even a very small one, invisible to the naked eye), a rash, an abrasion, a broken blister, or some other opening or weakness in the skin's epidermal barrier, and if that person is then exposed to infected blood or other biological fluids, in some cases there will be enough of a viral inoculation to cause infection.

In May 1987 the CDC, reversing its long-standing insistence that transmission by such means couldn't occur, finally reported three cases of just such transmission.[38] The three cases involved health care workers who came in skin contact with the blood of infected persons *without* needlestick exposure. The first case was that of a woman with chapped hands who "had a small amount of blood on her index finger for about 20 minutes before washing her hands." In the second case a woman who was wearing surgical gloves and eyeglasses, and who apparently had no open wounds, rashes, or sores, was splattered in the face with blood from an infected person, possibly getting some blood in her mouth as well. In the third case infected blood spilled on the hands and forearms of a woman who had no visible cuts or sores but had a rash on her ear that she might have touched. We are familiar with several other cases of this type, which have so far not been reported.

The practical implications of the clear-cut demonstration of this form of HIV transmission are ominous. First, it is likely that most such cases occur in situations where a person is not known to be infected with HIV. For example, a recent study of critically ill or severely injured patients brought to the emergency room at Johns Hopkins Hospital found that 6 out of 203, or 3%, were infected with HIV; in most instances, the study noted, emergency room personnel are not aware of HIV status while they are ministering to their patients, many of whom are bleeding or require medical procedures that expose health care workers to a patient's blood.[39] In addition, there are situations outside hospitals and health care facilities where bleeding is not rare; for example, in many sports events that involve a fair amount of contact, scrapes, cuts, and nosebleeds occur with some frequency. Is it possible to become infected with the AIDS virus in a touch football game, on the soccer field, while sliding into second base, or on the basketball court? In a word, yes. And until people who play such games do so wearing rubberized suits from head to toe (which, we hasten to add, we are not recommending), it is unfortunately true that a risk of inadvertent infection exists.

There is no way of quantifying the magnitude of this risk at present. But even if it is now very small, as the prevalence of HIV infection in the general population mounts, the risk of infection from nonsexual, non-drug-abuse, nontransfusion contact with blood will mount too. It makes for a scary situation.

3

CLINICAL FACTS
YOU NEED TO KNOW

At the present time we estimate that there are at least 3 million people in the United States who are infected with the AIDS virus. Clearly, though, only a small fraction of these people have progressed to outright cases of AIDS. In this chapter we will briefly describe the earlier stages of HIV infection and then discuss the likelihood that people currently in these stages will eventually develop the syndrome of AIDS. In addition, we will outline the basic principles (and pitfalls) of testing for infection with the AIDS virus, particularly focusing on the use and interpretation of tests designed to detect antibodies to the virus.

INITIAL INFECTION

In the first weeks immediately following infection with the AIDS virus, no matter what the form of transmission has been, there are usually no symptoms. This is particularly problematic because early symptoms provide a clue to the existence of virtually every other sexually transmitted disease, alerting the symptomatic person not only to seek medical assistance but also to abstain from sexual activity. In 10% to 25% of infected people a brief illness occurs two to five weeks after the AIDS virus invades the body, with symptoms that resemble either infectious mononucleosis ("mono") or the flu.[1] In these cases there is apt to be generalized achiness accompanied by fever, chills, itchy rashes, and swollen lymph nodes. Unfortunately, the nonspecific nature of the symptoms makes it quite unlikely that an affected individual will realize that he or she has been infected with the AIDS virus. In addition, even if an AIDS antibody test is done as part of the diagnostic evaluation of the illness, it will probably show a negative result because the immune system has not yet had time to respond to the infection by producing antibodies to the AIDS virus.

In a small number of cases initial infection is followed by meningitis (inflammation of the covering of the brain).[2] This usually produces an intense headache felt in the forehead or behind the eyes, as well as a stiff neck that can be painful if the head is bent forward. Other accompanying symptoms may include nausea and vomiting, fever, listlessness, and discomfort in bright light. Fortunately, this type of meningitis is not as serious as various types of bacterial meningitis and usually resolves spontaneously within a week.

Although these are noteworthy observations, it is important to emphasize the main point. *Most people do not have any symptoms of their initial infection with the AIDS virus; even when there are symptoms, these are of such a nonspecific nature that there's very little chance of recognizing what has actually happened.*

THE ASYMPTOMATIC CARRIER STATE

Following initial infection with the AIDS virus, most people feel perfectly healthy and have no idea that they are now infectious to others. This symptom-free period, which may persist for just a few months or for many years, is known as the asymptomatic carrier state. It is a time in which the carrier has live virus in his or her bloodstream but doesn't know it. Most asymptomatic carriers also have AIDS virus in various other body fluids, including semen, vaginal and cervical secretions, tears, breast milk, saliva, and sweat.[3]

It is important to realize that the virus present in asymptomatic carriers is exactly the same virus as the one that causes AIDS. It is not, as some people mistakenly think, a less virulent virus or a different, less dangerous strain of the AIDS virus. Thus, whenever this virus is transmitted to another person, no matter what the route of transmission, it has the potential to cause AIDS in the recipient, who also becomes a carrier of the infection with a lifelong ability to pass the AIDS virus to others. As Ho, Pomerantz, and Kaplan put it in the *New England Journal of Medicine,* "HIV persists in infected persons, who should be considered infected and infectious for life unless an effective therapy is developed."[4]

Why some people remain in the asymptomatic carrier

state for long periods of time, not developing any signs of illness, while others progress rather rapidly into symptomatic infection is not very clear at present. There is certainly the possibility that the underlying strength of the immune system is a primary determinant in this process. In other words, someone who has a stronger immune system that is in some fashion less susceptible to damage by the invading virus may be able to remain healthy longer than someone whose immune system is less powerful. Some scientists have theorized that people who are able to produce antibodies that somehow neutralize the AIDS virus may have a special advantage.[5] It is also possible, of course, that there is a certain threshold level of immune function that must be maintained in order to effectively fight off microbial assailants of many sorts. Thus, if a person has a "strong" immune system, the loss of as much as a third of his ordinary immune response may still leave him with adequate immune defense mechanisms. A person who starts off with a more marginal degree of immune competence, however, may find that the loss of a third of his immune capacity pushes him below the threshold required to combat invading organisms, resulting in a series of symptomatic infections that previously would have been turned away.

This concept is particularly important in light of evidence that more than 90% of people infected with the AIDS virus develop various types of immunologic damage within five years of developing antibodies.[6] Many investigators have found that a count of T-helper lymphocytes can be used as a rough index of immune competence: if the number is above 800 per milliliter of blood, it is an indication of a relatively unimpaired immune system; if the number drops below 400 per milliliter, it is a sign that the immune system has been significantly affected by the AIDS virus, and a harbinger of a quicker progression to symptomatic illness.[7] (Similarly, the T-helper lymphocyte count in persons with AIDS has been used as an indication of the relative state of their immune systems: if the count is under 200, for example, there is thought to be a much greater susceptibility to potentially fatal opportunistic infections.[8])

Other explanations have also been put forth to account for the conversion from asymptomatic carrier state to more overt illness. One of these points to the possibility of other infections (such as syphilis or hepatitis B) serving as cofactors that somehow activate the AIDS virus in asymptomatic carriers. Support for this theory comes from two different sources. First, there is clear-cut research showing that homosexual men in America are far more likely to have had past infections with hepatitis A and B, syphilis, and a variety of other microbial organisms than are American heterosexuals; furthermore, the prevalence of such infections among American homosexual men, though much higher than that found in American heterosexuals, is very similar to that in heterosexual African men and women.[9] Indeed, a number of parasitic and microbial diseases that are endemic in Africa and other tropical areas are known to impair the immune system,[10] which has led some experts to suggest that this may partly explain why heterosexually transmitted cases of AIDS are so common in Africa and Haiti.[11] Such coexistent microbial infections may act to speed up reproduction of the AIDS virus, to accelerate the invasion of virus particles into host tissues such as the brain or lungs, or to weaken the protection afforded by the immune system of the infected person. A second type of support for this infectious cofactor theory comes from recent laboratory studies. In part, such research has found that the AIDS virus is able to establish itself better in activated T-helper cells than in resting T cells—and this activation seems to be triggered by various viral infections, including the almost ubiquitous herpes simplex virus.[12] More important, a unique protein has been found in activated T cells that appears to control the multiplication of the AIDS virus in a manner somewhat like an on-off switch.[13]

Another proposed explanation for the progression from the symptom-free to the symptomatic stage is that repeated infection with the AIDS virus may play a role. With repeated infection—from numerous sexual contacts with an infected partner or partners over time, for example, or from repeated episodes of needle sharing with infected persons—the number of free virus particles in the bloodstream may be greatly increased, which may accelerate the rate of damage to T-4 helper lymphocytes and other cells that play a key role in immune defense mechanisms. Repeated HIV infection may also play a part in activating virus already present from previous infection.

SYMPTOMATIC CARRIERS

Once a person develops symptoms as a consequence of HIV infection, he or she crosses into a category known as AIDS-related complex (ARC). Definitions of ARC vary considerably, but typical symptoms include weight loss, fatigue, fever, night sweats, and diarrhea. In addition, there are sometimes accompanying minor infections such as oral thrush (candidiasis) or herpes zoster (shingles). Unfortunately, even though ARC is supposedly a set of symptoms and conditions that does not yet constitute full-blown AIDS, people can and do die from ARC if it follows a fulminant course. Inexplicably, the CDC has never precisely defined ARC or requested national reporting of this phase of HIV infection.[14]

There is a related category of HIV infection that some researchers believe is intermediate between the asymptomatic state and ARC, although others consider it more or less synonymous with ARC. This is a condition called PGL, or persistent generalized lymphadenopathy, which is marked by the appearance, unrelated to some other illness, of chronically swollen lymph nodes in several locations in the body. Although some homosexual men with PGL have seemed to remain relatively healthy for more than five years after developing it, many have progressed with time to ARC and AIDS, and virtually all have experienced deterioration in their immune functioning.[15]

Current research shows that once HIV-associated

symptoms begin to appear, a significant amount of damage to the immune system has already occurred, so there is a greater likelihood of progression to more advanced stages of HIV infection. However, there is considerable uncertainty about the timing of such progression. No one is exactly sure why some people with ARC develop AIDS within months while others seem to have a relatively more stable condition. There is some evidence, though, that in people with HIV infections the risk of developing AIDS is not constant over time but rather accelerates with the passage of time after infection.[16]

At present there is also considerable uncertainty about how many people infected with the AIDS virus will actually go on to develop AIDS. A few years ago estimates suggested that 20% to 30% of those infected would develop AIDS in a five-year period, but federal authorities were remarkably silent on what might happen after that time—leaving the impression in the minds of many that the ultimate risk associated with HIV infection was no worse than a one in three chance of AIDS, which of course translated into a one in three chance of death. Now there is much more pessimism about the outlook for HIV-infected persons. A research model developed in Germany projects that 75% of infected people will develop AIDS.[17] Some experts, in fact, have begun to glumly—and privately—predict that virtually everyone infected with this virus will eventually succumb to AIDS.[18] Even if the actuality is less severe than these predictions, it is still quite likely that a majority of infected persons will develop AIDS and die.

TESTING FOR HIV INFECTION

One of the key points in devising a successful prevention program is the identification of people who are already infected with the AIDS virus. Various methods are now available for this task. Because an understanding of such testing is pivotal to interpreting both our research findings, which will be described in the next chapter, and a number of issues that have major implications for prevention, we will turn now to an examination of tests for detecting HIV infection.

It would seem that the simplest, most direct way of detecting infection with the AIDS virus would be to attempt to isolate the virus from a sample of blood, a technique called a blood culture that is commonly used in medical diagnostics to identify bacterial infections. Unfortunately, viral cultures generally do not work as well as bacterial cultures, and though obtaining a positive culture for HIV provides unequivocal proof of infection, many infected people (including some with full-blown AIDS) do not have positive culture results.[19] HIV culture tests are also technically demanding and quite expensive, and they cannot be performed in most clinical laboratories.

Given the vagaries of trying to culture blood samples to determine if they are infected with HIV, it seems fortunate that a more useful screening method is available. This method involves detection of antibodies to HIV rather than detection of the infecting virus itself. (Antibodies are natural substances produced by the body's

41

immune system in response to any cell or organism it recognizes as "foreign" to the body; antibodies typically function by binding to the invader and neutralizing it in some fashion.)

The most commonly used HIV antibody screening test is known by the acronym ELISA, which stands for the technical name of the test, enzyme-linked immunosorbent assay. This test is relatively simple to perform as well as inexpensive (the actual cost is about \$2 or \$3, depending on the number of tests in a batch, although laboratories may charge patients \$25 or more). ELISA tests work by mixing serum with protein pieces of HIV in the presence of chemical reagents that cause a color reaction if HIV antibody is present. The intensity of the color reaction is read electronically by a special machine. The test was designed to be very sensitive, which means that it detects a very high percentage of blood samples in which HIV antibody is present.

According to various estimates, the sensitivity of the ELISA test under ideal testing conditions is approximately 98% to 99%,[20] which means that 1 or 2 samples out of every 100 that actually have HIV antibodies will be missed—a type of error known as a false negative result. (Unfortunately, testing is not always done under ideal conditions, as we will discuss in Chapter 5, so the actual test results may be somewhat less reliable.) However, in achieving this relatively high degree of sensitivity, the test errs somewhat more in its specificity—that is, it sometimes reacts to blood that does not contain HIV antibodies. These reactions, called false positives, are troublesome for a number of reasons that we will examine in detail later on—for example, they can have major repercussions for decisions about sexual relationships, childbearing, and medical care—but the key risk, of course, is that such errors can result in a misdiagnosis of infection with the AIDS virus, which will certainly be apt to have dire personal consequences. False positives seem to be most common in people who have received numerous blood transfusions and in women who have had several pregnancies, but they can occur in other cases too.

To guard against the high number of false positive readings that occur when only one ELISA test is used, it is standard practice in most laboratories to consider a test positive only if it is consistently positive with repeat ELISA testing and if the result is then confirmed by a more specific test such as the Western blot test. The Western blot is not used for the first phase of screening because it is relatively expensive ($50 to $75) and technically more demanding. Although considered more accurate than the ELISA test, the Western blot test is also not infallible. In one study of ELISA-positive blood donors who had positive HIV culture results, the Western blot was negative in 2 of 25 donors, which works out to a sensitivity of only 92%.[21] Other studies have also shown that the sensitivity of this test is far from perfect, although when used for confirmation on specimens that have already tested positive on ELISA screening, it has a high degree of accuracy.[22]

To put this all into perspective, it is important to realize that no medical test is 100% sensitive and 100% specific. In fact, for relative accuracy, current HIV antibody testing methods compare reasonably well to the broad range of laboratory tests. The problem is, of course, that an error in measuring someone's blood calcium or cholesterol level doesn't run the risk of stigmatizing that person or causing devastating emotional consequences. Even a false positive test for syphilis, which is not a medical rarity, is not likely to have the psychological, social, or economic consequences of a false positive test for HIV.

Testing for HIV antibody has another drawback in addition to the inherent inaccuracies of the methods currently employed. This problem, which may be far more serious from a functional point of view, is that people don't develop antibodies to HIV at the precise moment they're infected. In fact, a measurable antibody response to HIV infection may take three months to more than a year to occur,[23] although in the vast majority of people it seems to occur within the first six months following infection.[24]

The absence of a measurable antibody response in the early phases of HIV infection means that there is a time when ELISA testing will correctly show that a blood specimen doesn't contain antibody even though the blood is in fact infected with the AIDS virus. The implications of this "window of infectivity" problem for the safety of our blood supply and for personal strategies for evaluating whether it's safe to have sex with a new partner will be discussed further in Chapters 5 and 6.

Putting aside the problems of erroneous test results and the absence of an early antibody response, just what does it mean if a person tests seropositive for antibodies to the AIDS virus? According to the Institute of Medicine and National Academy of Sciences, "Any individual with antibodies confirmed by Western blot or other testing

44

should be considered to represent risk to unprotected sexual partners or to others through blood, sperm, or organ donations."[25] Similarly, a blue-ribbon Consensus Conference sponsored by the CDC and various other federal agencies concluded, "All persons who are antibody positive for HIV, whether they are symptom free or ill, must be considered to be potentially infectious to others by sexual transmission, by sharing of drug injection equipment, by childbearing, or by donation of blood, semen, or organs."[26]

These conclusions are in sharp contrast to positions taken by many individuals in 1985, when HIV antibody testing first came into widespread use. Then it was argued that the presence of the antibodies might only signal an exposure to the AIDS virus, just as a person who has a bout of measles develops antibodies while successfully fighting off the infection. Though this idea gained some temporary currency, especially among those who opposed the idea of widespread screening programs (including the screening of blood donors),[27] it was fortunately set aside as compelling evidence became available that the seropositive state is in effect synonymous with active infection.

It is likely, of course, that technological advances and greater understanding of the AIDS virus will lead to increasingly accurate second- and third-generation tests for identifying people infected with the AIDS virus. Procedures for measuring HIV antigen (protein portions of the AIDS virus capsule) that are already being tested carry some promise in this regard, especially since preliminary data suggest that in some cases they may succeed in detecting infection before measurable amounts

45

4

INFECTED HETEROSEXUALS: NEW EVIDENCE

In late 1985 our suspicion that infection with the AIDS virus was breaking out of the original high-risk groups led us to think about ways of testing this hypothesis. One of the options considered was a national probability survey of young adults that would provide descriptive data about their sexual behavior and correlate this information with the findings of blood tests for AIDS antibody status. This plan was abandoned for several different reasons. First, we believed that difficulties in obtaining the informed consent of potential study subjects would introduce considerable volunteer bias into the project and cloud the issue of whether we had a truly random sample. Second, we determined that the logistics of implementing this plan would be cumbersome since we would have to do interviews and blood tests in all fifty states to get a truly representative national sample. Third, the expense of an undertaking of this scope was prohibitive, especially since we had no federal funding to support such a project and very little prospect of obtaining any. Finally, we were led to believe that the CDC was considering sponsoring just such a study (although we recently learned that the project never really got started, in part because of political difficulties). We then looked at a number of variations on this approach that could answer the question we were raising in a less cumbersome, less expensive fashion.

RESEARCH DESIGN

One way to cut down expenses significantly was to conduct the interviews in just a few locations rather than in many different cities. It was important to do testing in several different regions of the country because results obtained in one location only—for instance, New York City or San Francisco—might be viewed as atypical and inapplicable to other areas. Thus, we decided to conduct our study in four large cities, two of which—New York and Los Angeles—were considered "high-risk" areas for AIDS, and two of which—St. Louis and Atlanta—were not.

We also decided that it made more sense to do a targeted study of two heterosexual populations that were distinctly different in terms of number of sex partners than to simply test a large group of heterosexuals without regard to sexual behavior patterns. Although we had discussed this idea for several months during the early and middle part of 1986, we were influenced strongly in this direction by the appearance of an important paper in the *Journal of the American Medical Association* in September of that year. This report, which was done by Alter and others under the auspices of the CDC, examined hepatitis B virus transmission in heterosexuals and found a strong correlation between the number of recent and lifetime sexual partners and the prevalence of hepatitis B infection.[1] The relevance of this observation to heterosexual transmission of the AIDS virus was especially clear since the group at highest risk for sexually transmitted hepatitis B is homosexual men.[2] Alter and her co-workers noted, "This study shows that for white heterosexuals the risk of acquiring HBV [hepatitis B virus] infection increases with increasing numbers of sexual partners and is independent of other risk factors known to be associated with acquiring HBV infection."[3] This finding was consistent with our working hypothesis that infection with the AIDS virus would be more common in heterosexuals with larger numbers of sex partners than in heterosexuals with a small number of partners.

We decided that the most efficient study design for us would be to compare two groups of sexually active heterosexuals: one group (the study group) in which each subject had had at least 6 different sex partners each year for the past five years, and the other group (the control group) made up entirely of people who had been in monogamous relationships for the preceding five years and reported no outside sexual activity whatsoever. The rationale for choosing the control group was clear: with no outside sex partners, persons in this group should not have had any sexual exposure to the AIDS virus unless the partner they thought had been monogamous had in fact been otherwise. Precisely how to quantify the selection criterion for annual number of sex partners for subjects in the study group was not so clear, however, and considerable thought was given to this subject before a decision was made. In the final analysis we relied heavily on sexual histories we had obtained from research subjects who participated in a number of projects at the Masters & Johnson Institute in the late 1970s and early 1980s; these histories indicated that fewer than 5% of sexually active heterosexual adults below the age of 40 had 6 or more sex partners in any given year.

Subjects aged 21 to 40 were recruited for potential participation in this project in a nonrandom, opportunistic manner (see Appendix B). For instance, married subjects were recruited in part through contacts in childbirth classes and church groups; cohabiting subjects were recruited through bulletin board announcements on more than a dozen university campuses; and single subjects were recruited through fliers distributed at singles bars, singles dances, and campus locations. In many instances recruitment was conducted by word of mouth and referrals from those who had already come in for screening. Such referrals were instrumental in permitting us to find an adequate sample of persons with numerous sex partners, since otherwise we would probably have had to screen more than 10,000 people to find 400 who met all our requirements for the study group.

In early 1987 we began screening people by use of a brief written questionnaire to select those who would ultimately make up our study sample. In order to eliminate the chance that potential subjects might have become HIV antibody-positive as a result of nonsexual transmission, we adopted the following exclusion criteria. Those screened were not informed of the exclusion criteria so that they wouldn't falsify their responses just to be selected for the study.

1. No blood transfusions received from 1977 on
2. No use of illicit drugs by injection
3. No homosexual or bisexual contact from 1977 on

In addition, people who worked in the health care field and might have been exposed to infected blood samples, biologic fluids, or tissue specimens were excluded from the study, although this criterion was not applied in the initial screening phase.

A total of 3,805 men and women completed the initial screening questionnaire. Of this group, 1,326 were married, 437 were cohabiting, and 2,042 were single. Of the 1,047 married persons who had been married for at least five years and met the exclusion criteria enumerated above, 568 (54.3%) claimed not to have had any sexual contact outside their marriage in the preceding five-year period, and 485 of these 568 were highly confident that their spouses had not been sexually unfaithful during their marriage.

Only 211 of the 437 persons who had been cohabiting with their current partners for at least five years also met the exclusion criteria. Of these 211 persons, 99 stated that they had not had any sex partners outside their primary relationship during the past five years. Of these 99, only 61 were highly confident that their partners had been sexually faithful during their relationship.

Of the 2,042 singles who were screened, 430 met all

the necessary criteria for selection to the study group.

In each of the four locations, 50 men and 50 women were selected for both the control group and the study group, giving a final sample size of 800. (Actually, 53 men and 53 women were selected for each group at each site. This was done so that we could eliminate data from any subject and have immediately available replacement data from a "substitute" subject in case of unanticipated problems, such as losing a blood specimen, discovering that a subject had misinformed us about one of the exclusion criteria, etc.) The control group of 400 consisted of 175 married men and 175 married women (generally participating without their spouses), as well as 25 cohabiting men and 25 cohabiting women. The study group of 400 consisted of 180 single men, 190 single women, 20 married men, and 10 married women. Descriptive information about the control group and the study group is provided in Table 4.1.

All subjects in the research program gave their informed consent to participation after listening to a tape-recorded explanation of the purposes and methods of the investigation and having an opportunity to ask questions. The tape recording emphasized the various steps that would be taken to safeguard the confidentiality of all research data, including the issuance of a code number known only to the subject, which would be used to ensure that data collection was done on an anonymous basis. A self-administered questionnaire identified only by the assigned code number was used to collect demographic information, health data, and information about sexual behavior over the preceding five years. The questionnaire also included a number of items designed to

TABLE 4.1
Characteristics of the Study Population

	CONTROL GROUP				STUDY GROUP			
	Men (N=200)		Women (N=200)		Men (N=200)		Women (N=200)	
Mean Age (Yrs.)	31.4		30.5		29.9		29.6	
Relationship Status[a]	#	%	#	%	#	%	#	%
Married	175	87.5	175	87.5	20	10.0	10	5.0
Divorced	0	—	0	—	14	7.0	26	13.0
Cohabiting	25	12.5	25	12.5	0	—	0	—
Single (not cohabiting)	0	—	0	—	180	90.0	190	95.0
Race								
White	181	90.5	178	89.0	179	89.5	177	88.5
Black	14	7.0	15	7.5	18	9.0	16	8.0
Hispanic	3	1.5	5	2.5	1	0.5	4	2.0
Other	2	1.0	2	1.0	2	1.0	3	1.5
Education								
Graduate degree	14	7.0	7	3.5	18	9.0	13	6.5
Some graduate study, no degree	8	4.0	6	3.0	14	7.0	17	8.5
College graduate	123	61.5	108	54.0	129	64.5	114	57.0
Some college, no degree	31	15.5	42	21.0	28	14.0	39	19.5
High school graduate	19	9.5	33	16.5	10	5.0	12	6.0
High school, no diploma	5	2.5	4	2.0	1	0.5	5	2.5
History of STD[b]	2	1.0	1	0.5	18	9.0	15	7.5

[a]Subjects were selected for the control group only if they had been in their current relationship (either marriage or cohabitation) for at least five years and had been entirely monogamous during that time. Study group subjects may be listed in more than one category (e.g., a subject may be both divorced and single), so numbers and percentages do not add up to 100.

[b]Subjects were asked by questionnaire if they had ever been diagnosed as having a venereal or sexually transmitted disease such as syphilis, gonorrhea, genital herpes, or chlamydia. Women who responded yes but stated during their interviews that the disease was a yeast infection, vaginitis, or monilia are not listed here as having a history of STD.

elicit subjects' attitudes towards AIDS. (This research questionnaire, along with the initial screening questionnaire, can be found in Appendix B.) After completing the questionnaire, each subject underwent a personal interview that typically lasted about thirty minutes. At the conclusion of the interview a blood sample was obtained to be tested for antibodies to the AIDS virus.

It must be emphasized again that all testing was done on an anonymous basis. Subjects were given a telephone number to call for the results of their blood tests *if they wished to do so.* It was made clear to them, however, that if they preferred not to obtain this information they were under no obligation to do so. It was also explained that since the researchers would have no means of identifying any study subject, the results of positive blood tests would not be reported to public health authorities or governmental agencies. Additionally, there was no way to break through the barrier of anonymity and report results to any study participant who didn't wish to know them. Finally, all subjects were informed that to provide maximum anonymity, the questionnaires used in the study and the master list of code numbers would be destroyed ninety days after completion of the project. (This was done to prevent the use of handwriting analysis or other potential identifying information in the event these materials were subpoenaed by a valid court order.)

All coded blood samples were tested for antibody to the AIDS virus using the ELISA test manufactured by Abbott Laboratories. Specimens that were repeatedly positive were then tested by the Western blot method for confirmation. Only specimens that tested positive for antibodies in both tests are reported here as positive.

FINDINGS

The average annual number of sex partners for the preceding five years in the study group was 11.5 for women and 9.8 for men. Approximately one-quarter of the women and one-fifth of the men in the study group averaged at least 15 different sex partners each year, as can be seen in Table 4.2. In contrast, the 400 subjects in the monogamous control group each reported only a single sex partner over the entire five-year period.

TABLE 4.2

Self-Reported Annual Number of Sex Partners for the Preceding Five Years for the Study Group,[a] by Gender

# OF PARTNERS	DISTRIBUTION OF STUDY GROUP BY YEAR									
	1982		1983		1984		1985		1986	
	#	%	#	%	#	%	#	%	#	%
Men										
6–9	95	47.5	98	49.0	94	47.0	98	49.0	97	48.5
10–14	65	32.5	62	31.0	64	32.0	66	33.0	63	31.5
15–19	37	18.5	37	18.5	39	19.5	33	16.5	36	18.0
20–24	2	1.0	1	0.5	2	1.0	2	1.0	3	1.5
≥25	1	0.5	2	1.0	1	0.5	1	0.5	1	0.5
Women										
6–9	91	45.5	90	45.0	94	47.0	94	47.0	92	46.0
10–14	62	31.0	62	31.0	56	28.0	54	27.0	60	30.0
15–19	40	20.0	39	19.5	43	21.5	41	20.5	40	20.0
20–24	5	2.5	6	3.0	4	2.0	7	3.5	6	3.0
≥25	2	1.0	3	1.5	3	1.5	4	2.0	2	1.0

[a]The study group consisted of 200 heterosexual men and 200 heterosexual women who reported having at least 6 sex partners annually for the past five years.

Among the 400 strictly monogamous men and women in our sample, only one man tested positive for antibodies to the AIDS virus. There was a strikingly higher prevalence of infection in the study group: 10 out of 200 men (5%) and 14 out of 200 women (7%) tested positive for HIV antibodies (see Table 4.3).* These differences were judged to be statistically significant since a chi-square analysis showed that the probability of such a discrepancy between the two groups occurring by chance alone was well under 1 in 100 ($p < .01$).

Since the hypothesis underlying our investigation was

TABLE 4.3
HIV Antibody Prevalence, Study Group Versus Control Group, by Gender[a]

HIV ANTIBODY STATUS	CONTROL GROUP		STUDY GROUP	
Men	#	%	#	%
Positive	1	0.5	10	5.0
Negative	199	99.5	190	95.0
Women				
Positive	0	—	14	7.0
Negative	200	100.0	186	93.0

[a]The control group consisted of 200 heterosexual men and 200 heterosexual women who had been in exclusively monogamous relationships for at least the past five years; the study group consisted of 200 heterosexual men and 200 heterosexual women who had averaged at least 6 sex partners a year for the preceding five years.

*So far as we knew, none of these people had been previously tested or were aware that they were seropositive.

that heterosexuals with the largest number of sexual partners would be most likely to be infected with the AIDS virus, we also examined the study subgroup that averaged more than 12 sex partners annually for the preceding five years (see Table 4.4). Not surprisingly, the prevalence of infection was even higher in this group: 14% (11 out of 80) of the women and 12% (7 out of 59) of the men in this category were seropositive. The difference between HIV antibody prevalence rates in these male and female subgroups and the remainder of the study group was also statistically significant ($p < .005$ in both cases).

The geographic distribution of cases of HIV infection was not particularly remarkable. The highest percentage of seropositive study subjects was found in the New York and Los Angeles areas (see Table 4.5), a finding in line with our expectations based on other reports of prevalence data.

More women with numerous sex partners had performed oral sex in the preceding year than had monoga-

---

TABLE 4.4
HIV Antibody Prevalence Rates in the Study Group, by Average Annual Number of Sex Partners for the Preceding Five Years and by Gender

	PREVALENCE RATE			
	Men		Women	
AVERAGE ANNUAL # OF PARTNERS	% Positive	# Positive/ # in Group	% Positive	# Positive/ # in Group
6–12	2.1	3/141	2.5	3/120
13+	11.9	7/59	13.8	11/80

TABLE 4.5
HIV Antibody Prevalence Rates for the Study Group, by Geographic Area

| | PREVALENCE RATE | | | |
| | Men | | Women | |
	% Positive	# Positive/ # in Group	% Positive	# Positive/ # in Group
New York	8.0	4/50	10.0	5/50
St. Louis	2.0	1/50	4.0	2/50
Atlanta	4.0	2/50	6.0	3/50
Los Angeles	6.0	3/50	8.0	4/50

TABLE 4.6
Self-Reported Participation in Various Types of Sexual Activity in the Preceding Twelve Months, Study Group Versus Control Group, by Gender

| | CONTROL GROUP | | | | STUDY GROUP | | | |
| | Men (N=200) | | Women (N=200) | | Men (N=200) | | Women (N=200) | |
TYPE OF ACTIVITY	#	%	#	%	#	%	#	%
Solitary masturbation to orgasm	176	88.0	154	77.0	183	91.5	163	81.5
Masturbation to orgasm by partner	26	13.0	168	84.0	28	14.0	156	78.0
Giving oral sex	85	42.5	147	73.5	108	54.0	192	96.0
Receiving oral sex	162	81.0	103	51.5	199	99.5	168	84.0
Vaginal intercourse	200	100.0	200	100.0	200	100.0	200	100.0
Anal intercourse	18	9.0	23	11.5	28	14.0	35	17.5

mous women (96% versus 73.5%), as shown in Table 4.6. Moreover, for those women in the overall sample who had performed oral sex on their partners in the preceding year (192 in the study group, 147 in the controls), there was a marked discrepancy in the frequency of engaging in this activity: on average, the women with numerous sexual partners performed oral sex twice as frequently as the monogamous women (see Table 4.7).

There was no meaningful correlation between the frequency of a woman's engaging in fellatio and the likelihood of infection with the AIDS virus: 4 of the 57 women who performed fellatio twelve times or more per month

---

TABLE 4.7
Self-Reported Average Monthly Frequencies for Various Types of Sexual Activity in the Preceding Twelve Months, Study Group Versus Control Group, by Gender

	AVERAGE MONTHLY FREQUENCY			
	Control Group		Study Group	
TYPE OF ACTIVITY	Men	Women	Men	Women
Solitary masturbation to orgasm	1.8	0.9	1.7	1.4
Masturbation to orgasm by partner	0.1	2.3	0.1	3.3
Giving oral sex	2.4	4.3	3.1	8.7
Receiving oral sex	3.6	1.9	6.6	5.5
Vaginal intercourse	8.5	9.8	9.7	10.8
Anal intercourse[a]	0.4	0.5	0.9	1.4

[a]Frequency figures for anal intercourse are only for subjects reporting participation in this activity (control group men N=18; control group women N=23; study group men N=28; study group women N=35); other figures show frequency for all 200 subjects in each subgroup of men and women, whether they reported participation in the activity or not.

were seropositive, while 3 of the 45 women who performed fellatio less than four times a month were seropositive.

It is noteworthy that substantially fewer men had performed cunnilingus in the preceding year than reported having had fellatio performed on them by their female partners. This discrepancy was present both in the control group, where 42.5% of the men had performed cunnilingus but 81% had experienced fellatio, and in the study group, where 54% of the men had engaged in cunnilingus and 99.5% had experienced fellatio. There was no link demonstrated between the HIV antibody status of men in the study group and their performance of oral sex: 6 out of 108 men who had performed cunnilingus were seropositive, compared to 4 out of the 92 who did not participate in cunnilingus.

Only a small minority of subjects in both groups had participated in anal intercourse in the preceding year. It is notable that this type of sexual activity was about 50% more prevalent among subjects with numerous sexual partners than among monogamous subjects (see Table 4.6). As Table 4.7 shows, for the female subjects who had engaged in anal sex, the frequency of this activity was about three times higher in the study group than in the control group. Of the 35 women in the study group who had a history of anal intercourse, 4 (11.4%) tested positive for HIV infection; of the 165 women who had no history of anal intercourse in the preceding year, 10 (6.1%) were seropositive. This difference was not statistically significant, however.

It is particularly notable that the self-reported average monthly frequencies of participation in vaginal intercourse are quite similar if we compare the men in the study group with the men in the control group and do the same for the women (see Table 4.7). The group frequencies for male and female masturbation are rather similar as well. However, the frequency of oral sex is decidedly higher in the men and women with numerous sexual partners. Men in this group reported engaging in fellatio almost twice as frequently as men in the control group, while women with numerous partners performed fellatio twice as often as their female counterparts in the control group. Similarly, women in the study group reported receiving cunnilingus almost three times as frequently as the women in monogamous relationships.

It is also particularly notable that less than 10% of the men and women who had numerous sex partners each year thought they might be exposing themselves to infection with the AIDS virus. Most were convinced that AIDS was not a problem among heterosexuals. Many also indicated with some confidence that they could avoid sexual contact with infected individuals by intuitively recognizing that those individuals were in a high-risk group. A few men and women pointed out that they avoided sexual relations with anyone known to be involved with drugs; several women noted that they steered away from men who they suspected or knew were bisexual.

In keeping with this general lack of concern about being at risk for infection with the AIDS virus, none of the 200 males in the study group had used condoms regularly during the preceding year. (About one-fifth of these men reported having used condoms on occasion but not routinely and consistently.) Only 6 of the 200 women in the study group (3%) routinely asked their partners to use condoms during vaginal intercourse, although 4 others stated that they asked for condom use during anal sex. Obviously this small number of women represented the distinct minority who did feel that there was a risk of being infected with the AIDS virus in heterosexual activity.

Of the total number of 848 people who participated in the project (48 of whom were "alternate" study subjects whose data were to be used only in the event that one of the 800 "official" subjects had to be disqualified), only 462 (54.5%) called to obtain the results of their blood tests. Though we can only speculate on why this number is so low, it fits with the idea that many people would rather not know whether they are infected with the AIDS virus.[4] As one woman said to us just after her blood sample was taken, "I hope you can learn something from this project—but I'm not going to call. If I'm infected, I'd rather not find out about it."

DISCUSSION

The striking difference in prevalence of HIV infection between the study and control groups is consistent with two points made by a number of authorities: AIDS infection is spreading beyond the original high-risk groups into the heterosexual population, and the risk of becoming infected with HIV is higher for people with more numerous sexual partners.[5] The latter point is particularly highlighted in our investigation by the striking prevalence of HIV infection in the members of our study population who averaged more than 12 sex partners annually: the prevalence rate was 14% in this subgroup of women and 12% in this subgroup of men.

While we can be reasonably confident of the strong link between sex with many partners and the risk of HIV infection, it is difficult to be certain of the precise risk of infection that is attributable to specific types of sexual activity. One reason for this is that those individuals in the study group who engaged in anal intercourse more than once or twice a year also, as a group, engaged in both oral-genital sex and penile-vaginal intercourse more frequently than the group that never participated in anal intercourse. Another confounding factor is that the people in the study group who engaged in anal intercourse most often also tended to be people with the largest numbers of sex partners. Thus, it is possible that the heightened risk of infection with the AIDS virus in this group is attributable primarily to more exposures rather than to exposure by a route of transmission with a greater likelihood of causing infection.

The fact that we found a higher prevalence of HIV infection in women with numerous sex partners than in men with numerous sex partners probably reflects two distinct realities of the pattern of sexual transmission of HIV today. First, women who have sex with many men are apt to have had one or more bisexual males among their partners even if they don't realize it. This, of course, increases their risk of being exposed to HIV infection. Second, because male IV drug abusers substantially outnumber female IV drug abusers, the likelihood is greater that a woman who has many sex partners may eventually have sexual contact with a man who became infected with the AIDS virus through drug use than it is for the reverse situation to occur. In addition, it should be realized that the generally higher prevalence of HIV infection in men than in women reported by most large screening programs (e.g., the antibody screening of military recruits and hospital admissions) primarily reflects the effect of including men with homosexual, bisexual, or drug abuse histories in these populations, while we made every effort to meticulously screen persons with such histories from our sample. Though there may certainly be other explanations that fit our findings, it seems to us that these are the most directly pertinent ones.

In order to put these findings in perspective, it is important to recognize the limitations of a study of this sort. Because our study population was not obtained by random sampling methods and did not closely match the general U.S. population in terms of socioeconomic status, educational background, and racial composition, our results cannot be easily generalized. Furthermore, since it is not clear at present what portion of the heterosexual population is as sexually active as our study group in terms of numbers of different sex partners, these data must certainly be interpreted with a degree of caution.

It should also be noted that the information on sexual behavior in this study was obtained retrospectively, meaning that its accuracy is largely dependent on participants' ability to recall their previous numbers of sex partners precisely and to estimate the frequency with which they engaged in various types of sexual activity. Though reliance on recall data is almost universal in sex research—the method was pioneered by Kinsey and his colleagues and has been followed by most other major investigators[6]—it would certainly have been preferable, had we had the financing and the time, to conduct a prospective study in which all subjects kept research logs listing the details of their sexual behavior on a daily basis. (Even this sort of prospective study is not error-free, of course; one problem is that subjects may change their patterns of sexual behavior in one direction or another because they know they are being studied.)

Despite these limitations, we believe this is an important study that has a number of strengths. So far as we know, it is the first large-scale research project attempting to correlate HIV infection in heterosexual men and women with a detailed analysis of sexual behavior. The fact that the study was conducted on a sizable nonclinical sample obtained in four locations in different regions of the country provides some confidence both in the statistical findings and in the degree to which the data reflect current trends of infection with the AIDS virus. (Clinical populations, such as patients attending sexually transmitted disease clinics, are much less useful for this type of research than nonclinical populations.) The large control group of exclusively monogamous heterosexual men and women is a particularly important feature of the study, since it allows us to compare not only rates of HIV infection in the two groups but differences in patterns of types and frequencies of sexual behavior that are especially informative.

One other aspect of this study should be noted. The

population we studied consisted mainly of ordinary, generally unremarkable middle-class men and women in their twenties and thirties—including teachers, repairmen, lawyers, secretaries, accountants, salesmen, waitresses, students, house painters, musicians, corporate executives, and some who were unemployed. In particular, we must point out that the 400 individuals who reported having sex with relatively large numbers of partners are not nymphomaniacs and satyrs; by and large they are single men and women who regard their sexuality as a healthy and fulfilling part of their lives. These people, who grew up during the sexual revolution, are not compulsively driven by the idea of having numerous sex partners for the sake of variety; rather, because they have difficulty finding a person with whom they can form a committed, one-to-one relationship, many of them engage in casual sex as a social act.

Here are comments from several people in the study group illustrating why they've chosen a nonmonogamous approach to sex:

> *A 33-year-old divorced woman:* I've always had an appetite for sex. Even while I was married I had an occasional fling. To me, sex is just a way of having fun and excitement—and it doesn't cost as much as lots of other exciting activities.

> *A 27-year-old male truck driver:* I'm on the road so much of the time that if I tried to stay faithful to someone, my sex life would be pretty sparse. Picking someone up in a bar or on the road isn't too hard, and it sure breaks up the monotony.

A 25-year-old female graduate student: I got started with a pretty active sex life when I was 15, and it's an important part of my life. I think that getting your clothes off and getting it on gives you a great insight into someone else's character.

A 32-year-old male stockbroker: Sex is my way of releasing tension. When you've been trying to drum up business all day and dealing with customers with a big smile, the tension builds up inside. At night I let it out with sex instead of getting bombed. And there are lots of gals around who are happy to hop into bed with me in return for dinner or a show.

In some instances, remaining single and uncommitted seems to be a lifestyle choice for these men and women. As one 28-year-old female attorney in our sample said, "I just don't have time right now to find a husband—I'm too busy trying to make partner at my firm." Other men and women also indicated that their educational and occupational goals made it difficult for them to think of marrying at this juncture in their lives. In other instances, being single was the by-product of one or more prior marriages that had fallen apart; 13% of the women and 7% of the men in our study group were divorced.

One of the most alarming findings in our study—and one that may surprise many people—is that few of the men and women engaging in sex with numerous partners were concerned about the risk of becoming infected with the AIDS virus. This lack of concern is expressed in behavioral terms by the minimal degree of change in their annual number of sex partners from 1982 to 1986 (see Table 4.2). Such nonchalance might have been understandable in 1983, when the epidemic was in its early stages, but the persistence of this attitude in 1987 strongly suggests that public health authorities have failed to impress the general public with the message that AIDS has broken out. Indeed, even warnings from the U.S. Surgeon General and other experts that sex with numerous partners is risky sex[7] seem to have been largely disregarded by the very segment of the heterosexual population they were intended to alert. This, in turn, creates new concerns: first, that the rate of spread of HIV infection will continue to climb relatively unchecked; and second, that repeated warnings do not by themselves necessarily result in the desired behavioral changes.

We do not suggest, of course, that either our study group or our control group is representative of the American young adult population. It is quite possible that as a result of concerns about AIDS, many heterosexual adults who are not in monogamous relationships have already become more cautious about sex (although in later chapters we will cite data from other studies that support the findings we present here). But the somewhat chilling conclusion we have reached is this: the AIDS virus has certainly established a beachhead in the ranks of heterosexuals, and because heterosexuals who have large numbers of sex partners are most likely to be infected, the odds are that the rate of spread among heterosexuals will now begin to escalate at a frightening pace.

5
HOW SAFE IS THE NATION'S BLOOD SUPPLY?

Since 1985 the American Red Cross, local blood banks, and various state and federal agencies have consistently issued public assurances that with the advent of routine testing for antibody to the AIDS virus, the nation's blood supply is now "virtually safe" from the risk of transfusion-transmitted AIDS. Strong statements have been used to allay the public's fears on this score particularly because in 1983 and 1984 many blood banks experienced a severe drop in numbers of blood donors due to a colossal but common misconception that the act of *donating* blood could somehow cause AIDS. Although attempts to correct this misconception were undertaken, they did not stress that people could only get AIDS by *receiving* blood, because many authorities in the field seem to have felt that such an educational campaign was fundamentally counterproductive. The problem was that it drew attention to the fact that transfusion-transmitted AIDS was a reality, and the blood banking industry preferred, for self-interested reasons, to minimize this point.[1]

The repeated statements that the nation's blood supply is now safe from the threat of AIDS generally echo

69

this one made by the Centers for Disease Control in 1987: "The risk of HIV transmission by transfusion was low, even before screening, and has been virtually eliminated by the routine screening of donated blood and plasma."[2] Language of this sort—the risk has been "virtually eliminated," the nation's blood supply is "virtually safe"—suggests to most intelligent observers that only a handful of cases of HIV infection are caused by transfusion each year. Regrettably, this impression and this claim are false. The fact that such information is widely disseminated, especially with such influential sponsorship, creates an alarming situation in which the general public is deceived.

DEFINING THE RISK

It is certainly true that the routine use of ELISA screening for blood donors has made the current situation far safer than it would otherwise be. It must be recognized, however, that any biomedical screening test suffers from certain sources of error—that is to say, it is not accurate 100% of the time. The ELISA test is no exception. Although it has a reasonably high degree of specificity as a screening test, it has a false negative rate of about 2%.[3] This means that given 100 blood samples known to contain antibody to the AIDS virus, the ELISA test will incorrectly report 2 as antibody-free. In fact, in ELISA tests of 88 people with full-blown cases of AIDS, 2 of them did not test positive for AIDS antibodies, giving a false negative rate of 2.3% in this most extremely ill population.[4] Similarly, in another study, 4 out of 69 AIDS patients had false negative ELISA tests, giving a false negative rate of 5.8%.[5] It is not inconceivable that the rate of false negatives may be somewhat higher in cases that have not progressed to the full clinical syndrome of AIDS.

Part of the problem has to do with the variability of ELISA tests made by different manufacturers in their capacity to detect a type of antibody called P-24 that is present in the relatively early stages of HIV infection. For instance, a study conducted by Alfred J. Saah, M.D., and his colleagues at the National Institute of Allergy and Infectious Diseases showed alarmingly high problems in precisely this type of early antibody detection, as well as great variability in the tests made by different manufacturers.[6] Specifically:

- The ELISA test made by Abbott Laboratories, which is the major supplier for the American Red Cross, failed to detect HIV antibody in 17 out of 30 positive specimens, for a false negative rate of 56.7%.

- The ELISA test made by another manufacturer failed to detect HIV antibody in 28 out of 30 positive specimens, for a false negative rate of 93.3%.

- The ELISA test made by Electro-Nucleonics, Inc., which is the primary supplier for the U.S. military's extensive blood testing program, failed to detect HIV antibody in 26 out of 30 positive specimens, for a false negative rate of 86.7%.

- The ELISA tests made by two other companies did considerably better than those mentioned above,

71

but each still failed to identify HIV antibody in 5 out
of 30 positive specimens, for a false negative rate of
16.6%.

Other studies have also reported a great deal of variability in the results yielded by different ELISA test kits.[7]
(The apparently low level of reliability found by Saah
and his colleagues in the ability of these kits to detect
early-stage HIV infection does not necessarily reflect the
overall accuracy of the kits in large-scale screening programs.)

In addition to the false negatives caused by the inherent limitations of the test method (e.g., the inability to
detect very low titers of antibody, or the presence in a
specimen of other substances that might bind or mask
HIV antibody), false negatives also occur because of various types of human error. To our knowledge, the frequency of such human-error false negatives has not been
examined in regard to AIDS antibody screening, but this
does not mean the problem is inconsequential. Just as
surgeons sometimes mistakenly sever a blood vessel or
leave a sponge inside a patient, and mail carriers sometimes deliver a letter to the wrong address, incorrect test
results can occur in a wide variety of circumstances, as
anyone familiar with laboratory operations will confirm:
for example, a technician uses testing reagents that are
outdated or neglects to add reagents to a tube when
doing a large number of tests together; a specimen gets
dropped, and a portion of the serum to be tested spills
out; a technician inadvertently mixes two serum specimens in the same test; a frozen serum sample is incom-
pletely thawed when it is tested; labels slip off tubes, or

code numbers are smeared, resulting in mistaken identification of the specimen and perhaps in the accidental switching of negative and positive test results. The possibility of such mishaps is necessarily somewhat greater in a laboratory that uses relatively inexperienced or poorly trained technicians or doesn't employ careful quality control standards, but the frightening reality is that even excellent laboratories have lapses in test performance when workers are under time pressure or when they are dealing with personal problems (including drug and alcohol abuse) or are otherwise stressed or just careless.[8]

These are not merely theoretical musings. According to a recent article in *Science,* 10 of the 19 laboratories that applied to the U.S. Army to conduct HIV antibody screening blood tests for military personnel had error rates of more than 5% on at least one occasion—which is especially remarkable, we might add, since they were apt to be at their most vigilant, knowing that the accuracy of their performance could result in a substantial and lucrative contract.[9] Even more startling, reports to the FDA in 1985 indicated that 13 units of blood known to contain HIV antibodies were released for transfusion through clerical error.[10]

These many sources of error take on a disturbing quality in light of the fact that current practice is not to retest initially negative specimens (due to expense, backup tests such as the Western blot are used only to confirm that a positive test is really positive). Thus, donated blood that is incorrectly certified as free of HIV infection as a result of a false negative ELISA test is automatically passed on to be used in transfusions.

Furthermore, it is a simple principle of immunology that an antibody response to infection is a *delayed* response. Measurable levels of antibodies do not appear in an infected person's system for weeks or months after an infection occurs. With the AIDS virus, whose properties are somewhat different from those of the common infectious viruses with which the medical community is familiar, a measurable antibody response may not occur for two to fourteen months after infection.[11] During this invisible "window of infectivity," donated blood will pass the ELISA test with flying colors but will transmit the AIDS virus to the recipient of the transfusion.

Admittedly, there is usually only a brief period of time, measured in weeks or months, when a person infected with HIV has not yet developed antibodies.[12] However, if HIV infection is currently being transmitted in the adult population at a rate of 500,000 new cases annually (which seems a reasonable estimate if we have gone from 1.5 million HIV-infected people in the U.S. in 1986 to more than 3 million today, as discussed in Chapter 1), this poses an ominous problem in terms of screening blood donors. If we assume that two-thirds of the new infections occur in homosexual and bisexual men and IV drug users, none of whom attempt to donate blood (though the latter assumption is unrealistic for a variety of reasons, it is useful since it simplifies our calculations and deliberately understates our results), then there are 166,667 new cases of HIV infection that do not fit these categories. If we further assume that 4% of this group will donate blood—an assumption in line with data on blood donor rates among U.S. adults[13]—there will be 6,667 people donating blood during the year of their initial infection (166,667 × .04 = 6,667). From this we can draw some inferences about the approximate number of infected units of blood that are passing undetected through the screening tests. Assume that each newly infected person has, on average, a two-month window of infectivity before becoming seropositive (that is, being detected by the ELISA test). This would mean that over a twelve-month period only one-sixth of the 6,667 people—about 1,111—will donate blood while in an antibody-negative but infected (and infective) state. HOWEVER, NONE OF THESE SPECIMENS WILL BE DETECTED AS CONTAGIOUS, SO THEY WILL BE UNWITTINGLY USED FOR TRANSFUSIONS. If the average window of infectivity is three months rather than two, the calculation works out to 1,667 people who will donate blood that is quite correctly certified as antibody-free but is in actuality carrying the deadly AIDS virus.

Similar calculations can be performed to examine the impact of ELISA false negatives on the safety of the nation's blood supply. First, we can conservatively assume that the estimate of 1.5 million Americans infected with HIV, which was made by various authorities in mid-1986, can now be modified to 2.5 million (for the spread of HIV certainly didn't stop or even slow down in late 1986). Second, on the assumption that two-thirds of this pool of infected persons consists of homosexual or bisexual men or IV drug users, of whom an estimated 95% will voluntarily exclude themselves from donating blood,[14] we are left with a group of 916,666 infected people who are potential blood donors (that is, 833,333 infected persons who are not homosexual or bisexual men or IV drug users, plus 83,333 persons who are). If only 3% of these people donate blood—an estimate that is lower than the blood donor rate in the under-65-year-old adult population—we can see that 27,500 units of infected blood will be donated in a year (916,666 × .03 = 27,500). With the ELISA test's 2% false negative rate, 550 of these units of HIV-infected blood will be incorrectly certified as safe (27,500 × .02), giving a total 1,661 units of HIV-infected blood (1,111 units from the "window of infectivity" problem plus 550 units from the false negatives) that will slip through the screening process. This calculation, which makes no allowance for other sources of error in ELISA testing, such as laboratory error, or for strains of HIV that are not detected by the ELISA test (see pp. 87–88), shows that the nation's blood supply is not, in fact, "virtually safe." There is a clear and imminent danger that the AIDS virus can be transmitted by any blood transfusion even in the era of AIDS screening.

To put this matter into perspective, it is helpful to realize that according to unpublished data provided by the American Blood Commission, there were about 18 million blood components transfused in 1984.[15] This represents, on average, two blood components derived from each unit of donated blood. Thus, the risk of becoming infected with HIV via transfusion of a single component of blood today, assuming the same number of transfusions annually, is about .0001845, or 1 in 5,418 (18,000,000 ÷ [1,661 × 2]). For a person who receives four blood components, the risk of becoming infected with the AIDS virus is 1 in 1,355.

While these numbers are certainly small, the risk they represent is not as insignificant as the blood banking industry or most medical authorities have implied. For instance, one recent report estimated that the current risk of an infected blood donation going undetected is 1 in 250,000.[16] The CDC, the Institute of Medicine, and the National Academy of Sciences have all issued very optimistic statements on the safety of the blood supply based on similar calculations[17]—but these projections are seriously flawed because they do not adequately allow for the infected blood that goes undetected before a measurable antibody response is present. In fact, the number of transfusion-associated HIV infections occurring today is not much different from the number occurring prior to the availability of the ELISA test for screening. For instance, according to an article in an American Medical Association monograph entitled *Information on AIDS for the Practicing Physician,*[18] there were theoretically about 4,000 cases of transfusion-transmitted AIDS that might result from transfusions received between 1977 and 1983. Another study estimated that there are now 12,000 people in the United States who acquired a transfusion-transmitted case of HIV infection between 1978 and 1984.[19] The truth is, then, that because the pool of HIV-infected persons has grown so rapidly beyond its pre-1985 size, the number of cases of transfusion-transmitted HIV infection will continue to grow unless a better method of blood donor screening is devised. Ideally, what we need is an efficient, inexpensive, and accurate HIV culture test to detect the virus rather than antibody to the virus, since this would eliminate the window-of-infectivity problem entirely and might conceivably cut down on the false negative rate as well.

DEALING WITH THE RISK

In light of the small but real risk of transfusion-transmitted HIV infection, what can be done? The best option at present is to donate blood to be frozen and stored for your personal use, which in many cases will obviate the need for transfusions from another person. This process, called autologous transfusion, has been recommended by a number of medical authorities,[20] although physicians only infrequently mention it to their patients even when there is elective surgery looming on the horizon.

In one large national multicenter study, it was found that only 5% of patients undergoing elective surgery and eligible for autologous transfusion actually predeposited their blood.[21] Notably, it was also found that 68% of the eligible patients who did not predonate blood would have completely avoided transfusions from other donors had they predeposited the number of red blood cell units ordered by their physicians. (These findings apply to short-term storage of blood for scheduled elective surgery rather than to the long-term frozen storage of predeposited blood as a general precautionary measure.)

Donating your blood for possible future use has several key advantages as well as several drawbacks or limitations. On the positive side, most people facing elective or nonemergency surgery will have enough notice of the possible need for blood transfusions to be able to donate several units in the months preceding the operation.

While there are certainly cases in which the amount of blood that can be donated is too small for the anticipated needs of such an operation, or where the underlying illness or a concurrent disease (such as severe anemia or infection) prevents the patient from donating blood even a few months before surgery, such situations are relatively infrequent. By insuring that any blood transfusion you receive during surgery (or convalescence from surgery) is your own blood, you completely eliminate the risk of contracting a transfusion-associated infection such as AIDS or the non-A, non-B form of hepatitis. You also completely eliminate the risk of an allergic transfusion reaction; since such reactions can at times be life-threatening (they can lead to hemolysis, kidney failure, and shock), there is an obvious benefit here as well. In fact, it is with good reason that a 1987 editorial in the prestigious *New England Journal of Medicine* was titled "The Patient's Blood Is the Safest Blood."[22]

Among the limitations of autologous transfusions, we might first mention a practical point. Even if you've had three or four units of your own blood frozen and stored, if you're in a major accident or require emergency surgery, there is no guarantee that you'll be brought to the hospital that is storing your blood or that there will be enough time to thaw the blood for your use. In addition, freezing and storing your own blood is an expensive proposition—it typically costs $500 to $1,000 to store three units of your blood for three years.

Despite these limitations, many people indicate that they would have a certain peace of mind if they knew that they'd donated their blood for possible future use. And most certainly, people facing elective surgery (or nonelective surgery that can be scheduled several months in advance) should give careful thought to predepositing their own blood in order to maximize the safety of any transfusions such surgery may require.

A different approach to the risk of transfusion-transmitted AIDS has gained some popularity recently but is based more on wishful thinking than on scientific validity. This is the practice, called directed donations, of choosing people to donate blood for your personal use. It operates on the thesis that people who are closely related to you or whose character you know well are not likely to have been infected with the AIDS virus. Regrettably, besides the fact that such individuals frequently don't match your blood type and so are unable to be of any help, there are no guarantees that your closest friend, whom you trust implicitly, is not bisexual or hasn't received a tainted blood transfusion or hasn't been a "closet" IV drug user. The intense pressure of the situation in which you are requesting blood donations may make it nearly impossible for your friends to refuse on grounds of membership in a high-risk group. Several authorities believe that there is no greater safety in directed donations than in simply accepting whatever blood is used by the local blood bank.

Since there are considerable variations in the blood banking policies of different hospitals, it is well worth inquiring to determine exactly what practices are permitted at your own institution. It may even be sensible in some cases to choose a hospital on the basis of whether or not it permits autologous transfusions.

It is also helpful to know that you can discuss a somewhat different form of autologous transfusion with your surgeon. During an operation the surgical team can collect as much of the blood you lose through bleeding as possible and retransfuse this blood into your body while surgery is still going on. Such a technique, which is known as intraoperative salvage and can even be used during emergency surgery, is a technically demanding but promising means of minimizing the risks of transfusion-transmitted infections.

6

CAN YOU CATCH AIDS FROM A TOILET SEAT?

The question posed by the title of this chapter is a reminder of current anxieties about an illness and a virus that are frightening in a very primeval way. Most people would like to believe that what they have been told about the AIDS epidemic by experts in newspapers and on carefully produced television specials is the whole unqualified story, but there is a lingering doubt that this is so. Wanting to be fair-minded, nondiscriminatory, and compassionate, people also understandably want to protect themselves and their children from becoming infected. So when they read in 1983 that AIDS was only transmitted by homosexual acts and subsequently learned this wasn't the case, they got nervous. When they read repeatedly that health care workers who came in contact with the blood and saliva of AIDS patients never became infected, they were reassured—until learning, in the spring of 1987, of several cases in which just such transmission occurred.[1] When they were told in 1985 that the blood supply was virtually safe from AIDS and then read about cases where infected units of blood slipped through the screening process,[2] or about two instances in which an infected organ was surgically transplanted to an unwary victim,[3] people became uncertain, confused, and more than a little unwilling to believe the voice of authority. In fact, even the neat, concise educational slogans about AIDS that are intended to be reassuring reminders to the world—like "You can't catch AIDS from a doorknob"—seem to some to be so oversimplified that they only provoke more anxiety.

In this chapter we will directly address some of the most difficult and widespread questions we've heard about the AIDS epidemic and the AIDS virus. In our answers we'll indicate just where the scientific uncertainties are and where commonsense responses to certain issues may be dead wrong.

Can you get AIDS from mosquitoes?

The final answer on this issue isn't available yet. Experiments have shown that mosquitoes do in fact ingest the AIDS virus and that the virus can live in mosquitoes for at least 48 hours.[4] The uncertainty comes from the lack of evidence that mosquitoes can actually *transmit* the virus. At the present time, for example, there is no evidence that the AIDS virus reproduces inside mosquitoes (or other insects), which would allow it to spread to the mosquito's salivary glands and thus be transmitted biologically in saliva the mosquito secretes as it feeds. But whether mosquitoes can be vectors of mechanical transmission of the AIDS virus is still an open question. Here is how an article in *Science* explained it:

> It is more difficult to categorically state that mechanical [as opposed to biological] transmission of AIDS does not happen. Mechanical transmission of virus

could theoretically occur if a mosquito, for example, was interrupted while feeding on an infected host, then flew to another person and injected a tiny portion of tainted blood.[5]

Most scientists feel that this is a farfetched possibility, particularly since the amount of blood "injected" in this manner would be exceedingly small, but it is not at all certain how much virus a person must be inoculated with in order for infection to result.[6]

Can the AIDS virus be transmitted in female-to-female sex?

Surprisingly, perhaps, the answer is yes. HIV has been identified by several investigators in vaginal secretions.[7] Either oral-genital contact, finger insertion in the vagina, or genital apposition (rubbing the female sex organs together) could result in transmission of the virus from an infected woman to her uninfected partner, but such transmission probably requires some sort of break in the skin. Although this is just a theoretical possibility, the absence of documentation of such cases may reflect the current low prevalence rates of HIV infection in lesbians more than it reflects a complete lack of risk associated with this form of sexual contact.

Why are hospital workers wearing rubber gloves even when they work with patients who don't have AIDS? Haven't the government experts said that there's no risk of infection from casual contact?

On July 23, 1987, it became mandatory for all health care institutions (including hospitals, nursing homes, and clinics) to comply in full with federal guidelines designed to protect workers against AIDS. Personnel such as nurses, physicians, and lab workers must now wear "barrier" protective devices—e.g., gloves, masks, and eye protection—when there is a possibility of coming in contact with any patient's blood or other body fluids. Failure to comply with these guidelines can result in fines of up to $10,000 for the institutions involved.

The reasons behind this policy change are complex but hinge largely on three realizations: it is impossible to know which patients are infected with HIV and which aren't; substantially higher numbers of people infected with the AIDS virus are being encountered in the health care system than had been suspected; and health care workers are not immune to infection with HIV through occupational exposure. According to the *American Medical News,* "This action comes in the wake of nine documented instances of AIDS cases among health care workers."[8]

Previously, many hospital officials and AIDS experts had downplayed the risks to health care workers in order to avoid an unseemly panic in which tens of thousands of workers might refuse to care for patients known or suspected to have AIDS. The belated recognition of the fact that there *is* a discernible risk involved—even though it may be much smaller than the risk of acquiring hepatitis B through occupational exposure—supports our contention that skin contact with infected biologic fluids can potentially result in infection.

Is there a possibility that a doctor could inadvertently transmit the AIDS virus from one patient to another by reusing contaminated equipment during an examination?

Although most physicians use disposable instruments for all invasive procedures—which completely eliminates such a risk—there are a few exceptions. For example, concern has recently been raised over the use of flexible sigmoidoscopes (for examining the rectum and colon) as an office procedure. Flexible sigmoidoscopes aren't built to tolerate the heat of the gas sterilization process recommended by the American Society for Gastrointestinal Endoscopy for instruments used on patients infected with HIV.[9] And according to Dr. Jerome Waye, chief of gastroenterology at Mount Sinai Hospital in New York, many office-based physicians are not employing other acceptable methods to sterilize these instruments. "They just scrub the sigmoidoscope, run some alcohol through it, and hang it up to dry for the next patient," he pointed out. Although the risk of patient-to-patient transmission of HIV may be low in such cases, it is certainly present. In fact, in 1985 the CDC issued a warning to the medical profession cautioning that since HIV is found in tears, it is important to disinfect instruments that come in direct contact with the external surface of the eye, as well as contact lenses used in trial fittings.[10]

Is it true that if a man has had a vasectomy, he can't transmit the AIDS virus?

No. Although a vasectomy prevents sperm from entering the male's ejaculate (by surgically severing the vas deferens, a pair of tubes that carry sperm from each testicle to the prostate), semen production and release are not eliminated (sperm cells only make up a small portion of semen, which is a liquid medium that transports the sperm). The AIDS virus isn't carried in sperm even in men who haven't had vasectomies; it is carried in semen, where it appears in white blood cells as well as in its "free"—or extracellular—state.

I had a blood transfusion in 1983. What are the chances that it may have been infected with the AIDS virus? Should I be tested now to see if I'm okay?

The use of HIV antibody testing to screen all blood donors didn't begin on a broad basis until the spring of 1985, so anyone who received a transfusion between 1977 and that time is potentially at risk. It's impossible to calculate the odds of having been given HIV-infected blood without knowing how many units of blood were transfused, but unless you received a large number of units, the chances are probably slim that you were infected—in part because the prevalence of infection in the general population was very low until recently. For example, it may be reassuring to know that in a recent study only 1 out of 2,343 people who received transfusions between January 1, 1977, and June 1, 1985, was found to be infected.[11] Nevertheless, if you are concerned about your personal situation, it is certainly appropriate to consider being tested now to get a definitive answer. It would be best to discuss this with your physician or with a counselor at a public health testing program to decide on how to proceed.

There have been some reports that there are several different types of virus that can cause AIDS besides HIV. Are they all detected by the screening tests?

It is true that at least two additional strains of the AIDS virus have been found. One, which was discovered in

West Africa, has caused AIDS in 17 people.[12] The other, discovered in Scandinavia, has also caused AIDS.[13] Both of these viruses are related to HIV but are genetically different in key ways. At present they are not usually detectable by the standard blood screening tests, and it is uncertain how rapidly these tests can be modified to identify all three viruses with any degree of accuracy. The existence of these additional viruses that can cause AIDS greatly complicates the task of developing a vaccine that will confer immunity against the disease.

Isn't it impossible to become infected unless you have more than one exposure to the virus?

Although multiple exposures of any sort are certainly apt to heighten the risk of infection, it's clear that a single exposure is all it takes for transmission to occur. For instance, there have been cases of HIV infection resulting from one-time artificial insemination with a donor's semen.[14] Likewise, we have seen a woman who was in a long-term, totally monogamous marriage and became seropositive four months after being raped. Instances of infection among health care workers from a single incident of being splashed with blood also confirm the fact that one exposure can result in HIV infection.[15]

Is it possible to catch AIDS from an infected kitchen worker or waiter?

As a practical matter, only if you share needles or have sex with that person. However, it is *theoretically* possible to be exposed in a restaurant under certain circumstances. For instance, if the chef cuts himself while preparing a dish that will be served cold (e.g., a salad, a sandwich) and his blood drips onto the food, infection could occur if whoever eats the food has a cut or ulceration of the lips or mouth that would give the virus a means of entry. Similarly, if you use a drinking glass or eating utensils that were previously used by an infected person and weren't cleaned properly, there is a small, as yet undetermined risk that you could be exposed to live, infectious virus from that person's saliva.

What are the chances that someone who's infected with the AIDS virus will actually develop a full-scale case of AIDS?

No one is certain of the answer right now. "Official" estimates during 1985 and 1986 were that 20% to 30% of infected individuals would develop AIDS within a five-year period, but those projections were based on very early readings of several research surveys. More recent studies have indicated that the numbers are probably far worse. For instance, one study done in Germany projects that as many as 75% of infected persons will eventually develop AIDS.[16] And according to *The New York Times,* "In private at least, many experts have begun to voice fear that in time, perhaps two decades or more, virtually every HIV-infected person will develop AIDS."[17] This is a particularly frightening prospect since no one with a full-scale case of AIDS has ever recovered. However, while it seems certain right now that many more infected people will progress to outright AIDS than had originally been hoped, it is certainly possible that those with the "best" immune reserves may fight the disease off for years or even for decades.

*Is there any reason for a person infected with the AIDS virus
to avoid sexual activity with another infected person?*

There is no definitive answer to this question. It would
seem at first glance that once you're infected, the damage is already done. However, some experts believe that
repeated episodes of reinfection may increase the
amount of virus in the body and thus may actually accelerate the progression of the infection. In light of this
uncertainty it would certainly seem prudent for infected
couples to adopt measures to minimize the risk of continuing reinfection.

*Is it possible that patterns of AIDS transmission will shift
so dramatically that we will eventually see the majority of
cases in heterosexuals?*

If the current epidemic goes on relatively unchecked—
and if there is no major success in the next year in
mounting an educational campaign that effectively moti-
vates people to change their sexual behavior—we believe
it is quite possible that just such a shift will occur. There
are several facts supporting this belief. First, AIDS is not
a "gay" disease. It is a viral infection that doesn't dis-
criminate in choosing its targets. Second, the AIDS virus
has already broken out into the heterosexual community, the primary conduit for this breakout probably having been the heterosexual partners of needle-sharing IV
drug abusers, and the secondary conduit the female sex
partners of bisexual men. Third, the immense size of the
pool of uninfected but potentially at-risk heterosexuals
is so much larger than the pool of homosexual and bisexual men, numerically speaking, that if no way of contain-

ing the rate of spread in the general population is found, the epidemic will explode in a manner that will make the numbers from 1981 to 1986 seem tame. Under these circumstances we would expect that by 1993 over a quarter of new cases of AIDS will occur in heterosexuals who are not IV drug users. By the turn of the century more than half of AIDS cases will be in the heterosexual population.

Do women have any special symptoms that may be clues to infection with the AIDS virus?

According to a recent study, the combination of severe, treatment-resistant, chronic vaginal candidiasis (sometimes called monilial vaginitis or a "fungus" or "yeast" infection) and oral thrush raises a distinct possibility that an underlying HIV infection may be the cause.[18] Thrush, a fungus infection of the mouth caused by *Candida albicans,* typically appears as white plaques or patches on the tongue, the gums, the palate, and even the corners of the lips. Vaginal candidiasis, or monilial infection, typically produces a thick, whitish, cheesy vaginal discharge as well as intense itching of the vulva. It is relatively common in women with diabetes and women who take antibiotics or birth control pills; these women need not be concerned if they have difficulty treating their candidiasis, since only *unexplained* candidiasis appears to be a risk factor for HIV infection.

Isn't it true that the AIDS virus only appears in the genital secretions of women while they're menstruating and that there's no risk of infection at other times because there's no bleeding?

91

This idea is erroneous. The AIDS virus appears in the cervical secretions of women throughout the menstrual cycle, not just during the days of menstrual flow.[19] In fact, the virus may not always be carried by blood cells— it may actually infect certain cells in the genital region and enter genital secretions by some local rather than blood-borne mechanism.

Is it true that "natural" condoms are less effective in blocking the AIDS virus than synthetic condoms?

Natural condoms are made from sheep intestinal membrane. Some concern over possible leakage has been voiced by various authorities, but there is no firm answer available just yet. One study that tested various types of condom for effectiveness in blocking hepatitis B antigen particles showed that the only natural condom tested did allow these particles to leak through whereas the synthetic condoms did not.[20] On the other hand, another study that used the AIDS virus in testing condoms did not find any evidence of leakage with natural condoms, although the number tested was admittedly small.[21] (For a more detailed discussion of the safety of condoms, see Chapter 7.)

Can you catch AIDS from a toilet seat?

The press has had a field day with questions of this sort. The derisive impression they are apt to give is that anyone asking such a question has an antediluvian, unenlightened attitude towards AIDS, since the notion has got to be wrong. Yet there is a certain undeniable fascination with this issue—and an equally undeniable reality to the answer we must give.

Although it is clear that if such a mode of transmission has ever happened, it must be an exceptionally rare occurrence, the fact is that it is theoretically possible to become infected with the AIDS virus from skin contact with a contaminated toilet seat (or any other contaminated surface). This alarming conclusion is based on research published in 1986 in the *Journal of the American Medical Association*[22] in which it was shown that the AIDS virus retains its infectivity for more than three days in dried blood kept at room temperature. (In a liquid state, "infectious virus survived longer than 15 days at room temperature."[23]) Though these experiments were conducted on highly concentrated virus samples that greatly exceeded the concentrations apt to be present in the biological fluids of infected patients, the fact of extended infectivity of the virus in dried blood (or other dried liquids) is plainly apparent. Thus, if infected blood (from a cut, scrape, ulcer, blister, or rash on the buttocks) or infected semen (either dripped from the penis or spilled from a condom) is inadvertently left on a toilet seat and someone who comes in contact with this material also happens to have a break in the skin at the point of contact, the virus may enter the body and infection may occur.

Much the same mechanism of infection may have been involved in the cases of two laboratory workers who were accidentally infected with HIV, apparently through spills of highly concentrated solutions of virus-containing material.[24] While the CDC was insisting emphatically that such infections were a theoretical risk only and had never happened in real life, they actually knew about one of these cases for over a year before they released the information to the public.[25]

7

SEXUAL CHOICES
IN THE AGE OF AIDS

Unless there is a remarkable and currently unanticipated breakthrough such as the development of a vaccine to prevent infection with the AIDS virus or the discovery of a cure for AIDS, we must all face the realities that the AIDS epidemic brings to our world. More than anything, this calls for making responsible, informed choices about our sexual behavior. In this chapter, we will discuss various aspects of sexual behavior in relation to the risk of contracting the AIDS virus.

ABSTINENCE

Although the choice does not have much appeal to most adults, there is something to be said for a deliberate decision to abstain from sexual activity as a means of completely avoiding the risks of sexual exposure to the AIDS virus. To serve this purpose, though, abstinence can't be a part-time proposition: it must become, in effect, a way of life. Clearly, choosing abstinence (as a cognitive act) and being completely abstinent (as a behavioral act) are not the same: even among Catholic priests, whose clerical vows impose lifelong celibacy, there have been more than a few cases of AIDS.[1]

Our experience over the years suggests that in general women seem to find abstinence an easier choice than do men. At least at this stage of the AIDS epidemic, this pattern continues to be borne out: our impression is that more single heterosexual women than unmarried heterosexual men are choosing abstinence. Without delving into the specific reasons behind this difference—which we believe are more culturally determined than biologically based—we will simply point out that the reasons for deciding to abstain from sex at a given time in one's life are apt to be particularly complex. When the decision is made in relation to AIDS, the common denominator for both genders seems to be fear, as shown by comments from several people we've interviewed who have chosen this option.

A 33-year-old recently divorced woman: All the news stories about AIDS still affecting mainly homosexuals, bisexuals, and addicts don't convince me. This disease is a killer, not just something you treat discreetly at your doctor's office with a shot of penicillin. Perhaps if I meet the right person I'll change my mind, but for now it's a relief to know that sex—except masturbation—is completely off limits.

A 21-year-old single male college student: I used to think that AIDS was some sort of rare, exotic illness that would never touch the people I know. I got a rude awakening when two classmates of mine found out that they're infected. To me, postponing sex for a few years sounds safe—like not going sailing in the middle of a storm. When the storm is over, then I'll be ready to sail.

A 26-year-old never-married woman: Let's face it—sex just isn't the most important thing in life. I'm certainly not opposed to sex, and I used to enjoy sex, but right now the sanest choice for me is no sex at all. No sex, no worries. No sex, no AIDS. It's really a very simple equation, isn't it?

A 23-year-old single nurse: I resisted jumping into bed with guys when I was a teenager and when I was in college. I suppose then I just wasn't ready. Now I'm ready, but I'm frightened too. So I'm not going to change my mind until I meet the man I'll marry. I guess there's something to be said for good old-fashioned virginity.

Abstinence is not an option being chosen exclusively by heterosexuals. A number of gay men have told us that they are reluctantly choosing abstinence rather than risk the high odds of exposure to AIDS during sex with other men. Here are two representative comments:

A 34-year-old gay male: I became alarmed by the news stories about AIDS in 1983 or 1984. It was clear to me that I was in the "official" highest risk group, and this was confirmed when a number of friends of mine came down with AIDS and died. Now, I may not be a genius, but I was smart enough to know that I don't want to trust my life to a condom. So the only sensible choices seemed to be: settle down in a one-on-one relationship with someone who's healthy, or give up sex. Giving up sex was simpler. It didn't really complicate my life. And I have no illusions about being celibate—it's a way of staying worry-free and staying alive.

97

A 27-year-old gay male: Gay pride is a great sentiment when there's something to be proud of, but being gay is nothing like that today. Not only is there that constant gnawing fear inside—"Was that guy really okay?"—and worries about losing your job, your apartment, and your sanity, but you have to wonder what it says about the intelligence of gays who keep going to bars, bathhouses, and parties with no particular precautions about sex. I'm no kamikaze. Being asexual for a while is better than the alternative.

We have also spoken with gay men who chose abstinence only after first trying to switch over to a heterosexual life. Most of these men, who had been exclusively or almost exclusively homosexual, were disappointed with the attempt to convert to heterosexual activity. (In contrast, we have seen many bisexual men who seem to have made a shift to exclusive heterosexual sex relatively easily.)

SAFE SEX

There is one set of circumstances under which all forms of sexual activity can be considered totally and completely safe from the standpoint of exposure to the AIDS virus. This is, of course, a relationship—either heterosexual or homosexual—where both partners have had no prior sexual contacts with anyone else and have not been exposed to the AIDS virus by nonsexual means. Although couples whose sexual histories are so exclusive may have been relatively rare in the past few decades, it is very possible that the strong comfort and appeal of absolute certainty in terms of worries about AIDS will make this type of sexual biography more common in the future.

One of the pragmatic questions that arises in regard to such relationships, and that will recur repeatedly at later points in this discussion, is how to be certain that your partner is telling the truth about his or her sexual past. The issue is not as simple as it might first seem to be. For one thing, judging from our experience with couples both clinically and in research, people are more apt to engage in some form of deception about their sexual biographies than they are to tell all. This tendency is probably compounded when an issue as volatile as possible previous exposure to the AIDS virus comes into play. Indeed, it is not difficult to imagine circumstances in which revealing one's sexual history to a partner could precipitate the breakup of a relationship, or at least seriously undermine the trust of that relationship.

Consider, for example, a young man in his early twenties who has been dating a woman for more than three years and has now become engaged to her. They have not previously had sexual intercourse, and they are both, heterosexually speaking, virgins. The man, however, had a brief homosexual relationship in his freshman year of college, involving only a handful of sexual encounters. He is certainly at risk for being infected with the AIDS virus. After wrestling with his conscience on the matter, he decides with great difficulty to tell his fiancée of these past encounters. On learning this news, she becomes so distraught that she breaks off their engagement. This situation is certainly possible, though more often than not, in our experience, it would play out differently: the typical man with this sort of sexual history would keep the information to himself, leaving his fiancée to believe that he is as inexperienced as she is. In either case, the consequences are dismaying.

Not very long ago it was reasonably accepted and even expected etiquette in most social circles for the great majority of young adults to have been sexually active prior to meeting the person they would decide to marry. Today the accepted etiquette is changing drastically as concerns over AIDS mount. While this certainly doesn't mean that people who have already been sexually active wish they hadn't been—in fact, relatively few single, never-married adults seem to want to be sexually inexperienced—it does create a new set of pressures when they decide it's time to marry. Judging from interviews we've conducted with several hundred college students, a sizable number of males and females will lie to a prospective spouse about their past sex lives. Few of them will claim to be totally inexperienced sexually, but many will minimize the number of sexual partners they've had or misstate the extent of their sexual experience. Some who will tell a prospective spouse that they have had previous sexual experiences will nevertheless lie about the consistency of condom use in these encounters. Substantial numbers of women will—certainly understandably—refuse to tell a partner about having been raped or having been the victim of incest. Men will be particularly apt to hide information about past homosexual experiences and sex with prostitutes.

What this means is that it is difficult to be certain

about the truthfulness of what someone else tells you about his or her sexual past. For this reason, even couples who are deeply in love, plan to marry, and have no reason to doubt each other's claims of no prior sexual contacts should probably consider being tested for antibodies to the AIDS virus. Though this sort of testing may provide only a low yield of positive results, it may be advisable because it can detect cases where infection with the virus has occurred through nonsexual as well as sexual means.

TESTING FOR SAFE SEX

While the risk of infection with the AIDS virus is greater among people who have had numerous sex partners than among those who have had few, *anyone* with prior sexual experience, however limited, must be regarded as a potential asymptomatic carrier of the virus. Likewise, anyone who has injected illicit drugs or received a transfusion in the preceding decade must be regarded as a potential carrier of the AIDS virus. Since there are now some 3 million HIV-infected Americans—most of whom, as we've said before, do not realize that they are infected and contagious to others—it should be a matter of utmost concern to anyone entering a new relationship to ascertain that a prospective partner is *not* infected before physical intimacy passes the stage of snuggling. Because infection with the AIDS virus cannot be detected from a person's appearance, and because personal disclaimers,

101

no matter how seemingly heartfelt and sincere, cannot reliably indicate freedom from infection, a more objective means of evaluation is required.

As a practical matter (albeit a cumbersome one), the only way to achieve a high degree of certainty at present is for both persons in the relationship to jointly agree to antibody testing before beginning any sexual activity. For the most stringent and conclusive assessment currently available, each person should first have an antibody screening test (such as the ELISA), to be followed by a more definitive test (such as the Western blot) in the event that the first test is even weakly positive. This minimizes—but does not completely eliminate—the possibility of false positive results. Then the couple should abstain from sexual activity with each other or with any other partner for a six-month period, at which time they should again be tested for antibodies to the AIDS virus. (The purpose of retesting after six months is to exclude the small but real number of cases in which the initial test occurs too soon after infection for detectable quantities of antibody to be in circulation.) With negative antibody tests in both partners at both testing times, and with an absolute commitment to remaining sexually monogamous, the couple can have the highest possible degree of confidence that there is no risk of contracting sexually transmitted AIDS. (It is of course possible that even if a couple undergoes this sort of double testing and remains absolutely monogamous, one of them could still be infected with the AIDS virus by nonsexual means. In this event, the virus could certainly be transmitted sexually to the other partner.)

Most couples will probably not be willing to abstain

from sexual activity for the six-month waiting period suggested above. It is, after all, an easy way to lose one's ardor—to replace passion with the cold, calculated precision of a scientific protocol. Furthermore, our sexual urges are not as likely to be ruled by temperate reason as, say, our willingness to wear a seatbelt in a car. And although wearing a seatbelt doesn't generally interfere with getting to our destination or using the car in almost any manner we choose, and certainly doesn't result in a six-month delay, many people deliberately disdain seatbelts even where it's a clear violation of the law (and of common sense about personal safety) not to use them. So the chances that large numbers of people will adopt the stringent double-testing conditions outlined above are slim indeed.

For this reason, we offer an alternative, slightly less reliable but still highly valid method of double-testing that permits sexual activity to commence promptly after the results of the initial antibody tests are received. If both partners' initial tests are negative, they can engage in sexual activity with the proviso that it involve absolutely consistent use of a condom during any episode of either vaginal intercourse or fellatio, as well as total abstinence from anal sex. Now, as we will discuss in more detail shortly, the use of a condom is not at all foolproof in preventing the transmission of the AIDS virus. But it will reduce the risk of exposure to the virus, not only when it is completely effective as a mechanical barrier, but even if it leaks—for in all probability the defective device still greatly reduces the number of virus particles to which the partner is exposed. Thus, in a situation that begins with one round of antibody testing—which may

detect, based on current scientific estimates, approximately 98% of infected persons—the use of a condom makes the risk much lower than it would otherwise be. Needless to say, if condoms are not used consistently, the risk is somewhat higher.

There are two particular areas of vulnerability in the testing approaches just described. Both hinge on the issue of trust. First, assuming you and your partner have both agreed to be tested, how confident can you be that you are going to be accurately informed of your partner's test result? Second, even if both of you have negative tests, how certain can you be that your partner isn't having sexual contact with someone else, thus potentially becoming infected from an affair that you don't know about?

The need to be sure that your partner has in fact been tested and that you can verify the results is not just a theoretical one that can be lightly set aside. For one thing, there are malicious, greedy businesses already in operation selling people (mostly men) bogus "certi-fied-AIDS-free" identification cards. (In some cases, the purchaser realizes he is getting a phony document; in other cases, the purchaser gives a blood sample and is charged a fee for a blood test that is never done, so that he or she is under the impression that the ID card or document is accurate.) Such ventures are fundamentally different from companies that actually perform the testing they sell (sometimes with accuracy, sometimes not), but it is quite difficult for the typical consumer to check out the operations and track record of private businesses in this area. We also know of cases in which people, including prostitutes, have forged official-looking letters

from physicians or laboratories stating that they were tested for AIDS and the results were negative. Prostitutes have an obvious economic incentive for such a ploy; in several instances we've encountered, men have used such letters in attempts at picking women up in bars. Furthermore, there are thousands of people who know that they're infected and are deliberately hiding this information from their sex partners. Some of them, having already gone through testing procedures, may be smart enough to know how to fake it (with regard to sham testing and "reporting") convincingly enough that an unwary partner will be fooled.

Beyond these cases of more or less preplanned, deliberate deception looms a much larger category. Here we include many ordinary, straightforward people who are genuinely shocked to discover that they've tested positive for antibodies to the AIDS virus. Some of them are so distraught that they completely deny the accuracy of the report. ("It must've been a mistake in the lab; maybe they mixed up my blood sample with someone else's.") Others simply deny the reality of the situation. ("It just can't be. I feel perfectly well—I *know* nothing's wrong with me.") Still others refuse to believe that they could be infectious to someone else. ("The antibodies in my blood mean that I was able to fight off the virus, not that I'm infected or that I could make anyone sick.") And others, even after they've been counseled and even realizing the implications of their infection, choose to hide the truth from current or future sex partners. This may be the most dangerous group of all. And it is in this group that we find some who will hide their actual test results from their partners, claiming that "the test was

okay"—and creating a clear potential for further spread of the virus.

Without belaboring the darker side of the human soul that permits such deception (and subsequent harm), it is useful to point out possible ways of avoiding these problems. For instance, a couple—either heterosexual or homosexual—can go to a physician for HIV testing, as millions have in the past for premarital testing, and instruct the physician that the test results are to be discussed openly with both of them. In some instances the physician may request that they sign a consent form authorizing such a discussion, since it involves, in effect, a waiver of personal privacy, but this is a simple issue. Another possibility is to use a clinic or public health facility that permits anonymous testing. In this situation the partners exchange code numbers so that each can call the testing office and receive the other's results. (Of course, this approach won't work if you can't verify that the tested blood sample and the code number actually belonged to your partner. Although this probably sounds somewhat farfetched, anyone familiar with drug-testing programs knows that there have frequently been attempts to substitute a "clean" urine specimen for one that will test positive for illegal substances.) Finally, it is possible in some locations to go directly to a university-run or hospital-based laboratory for confidential testing. If both partners instruct the laboratory to send their test results to them by certified mail in a single envelope, they can open the document together to see the lab report on each test.

The second type of vulnerability in the testing strategy we've suggested involves the trust implicit in believing

that your partner will be absolutely monogamous once the testing has been completed (or during the six-month interval between the first and second tests). Unfortunately, assumptions about sexual fidelity can be dangerous to your health. For example, in screening people for participation in the study described in Chapter 4, we found that among 785 married men between the ages of 20 and 40, 44.3% had had at least one extramarital sexual partner in the preceding five years. Among 541 married women we screened, 32.3% had had extramarital sex in the same five-year period. These figures are similar to data from other investigations.

Kinsey and his co-workers estimated in 1948 that half of all married males in their sample had had extramarital coitus; in their 1953 report Kinsey's group noted that by age 40, 26% of married women had been extramaritally involved at least once.[2] In 1975 a survey conducted by *Redbook* reported that 38% of married women aged 35 to 39 had extramarital sexual experience.[3] In 1983 Blumstein and Schwartz[4] found that 26% of husbands and 21% of wives in their sample had been nonmonogamous since the start of their relationship; among their sample group of unmarried people living together, 33% of the males and 30% of the females had not been monogamous. Blumstein and Schwartz note that marriage seems to make people more deceptive about their sexual behavior. They also observe, *"A couple can never be completely sure that their relationship will remain monogamous. Ten years of monogamy does not mean the eleventh is safe."* (Among gay men in long-term relationships, 82% had outside sex, and for lesbians the corresponding figure was 28%, according to the same study.)

It is certainly correct to point out that these early data were collected, by and large, before the AIDS epidemic and may not be completely applicable today as awareness of the risk of AIDS increases. Nevertheless, government statistics on other sexually transmitted diseases such as syphilis, which show increased numbers in 1987 compared to prior periods, do not point to a drop in nonmonogamous behavior among heterosexuals.[5] Likewise, the findings on current patterns of sexual behavior that we discussed in Chapter 4 and will also consider in the next chapter do not give much credence to the wishful notion that most heterosexuals have significantly modified their sex lives in response to the threat of AIDS. Indeed, although there has been much made of the distinct decrease in unsafe sex among gay men—including the practice of anonymous sex with multiple partners—at least some research suggests that this may have been a temporary change largely limited to a few metropolitan areas.[6]

For these reasons it is important to realize that the promise of safe sex offered by the double-testing procedure outlined here is only as good as the behavioral commitment to that objective. Testing only gives a snapshot of evidence about your condition at a particular point in time. If you are uninfected and you jeopardize your health status by having sex outside the "safe" relationship, you also potentially jeopardize the health of your partner, who innocently trusts in your common sense and sense of fair play. But the reality is, sadly, that the forbidden fruit is often more appealing than what is readily accessible, so it is virtually certain that even as the

numbers mount in the AIDS epidemic, millions of people will continue to follow libidinal urges that put them directly at risk of being infected with the AIDS virus.

There is no specific, foolproof solution we can offer here. While we are not suggesting that extrarelationship sex is always morally wrong, it seems reasonable to make the following points:

1. If you suspect that your partner has been sexually active with someone else, talk about your concern and find out what he or she has to say.

2. If your partner denies having extrarelationship sex and you aren't satisfied, consider asking your partner to be tested again.

3. Before embarking on any form of nonmonogamous sex, think carefully about the risks you're running—for your partner as well as yourself.

4. If the prospect of sex outside your primary relationship is so compelling that you can't put it out of your mind, consider having your prospective partner undergo testing to confirm that he or she isn't infected with the AIDS virus. If he or she refuses, our best advice is to head straight for the door.

There is one more cautionary note that we should add here. Recently, a number of entrepreneurs have hit upon an idea that sounds like an easy, straightforward way of simultaneously capitalizing on people's fears of AIDS and providing a useful public service. They have organized so-called AIDS-free singles groups that for a monthly or annual fee provide periodic HIV testing and expect members to have sexual contact solely with other group members (and avoid IV drug abuse). The theory behind this approach is simple: if you can prevent exposure to the virus by not doing drugs and by limiting your sexual contacts to people who are not infected, you can't come down with AIDS. In a sense this is an extension of the double-testing monogamous strategy we've recommended here, but instead of monogamy it calls for loyalty and sexual fidelity to a group. Unfortunately, there is apt to be a huge gap between theory and practice with such clubs and organizations. Referring to the diminishing probability that people in such clubs or groups will consistently conform to the rules, a physician at the AMA observes, "It's like people who go on diets: they're able to sustain it for a while, but then their commitment wanes."7

The bottom line here is that testing programs aimed at fostering truly safe sex do not provide an ironclad, unassailable guarantee. What is required for assurance that no sexual exposure to the AIDS virus can occur is for two partners to be accurately tested on two occasions, at least six months apart, and then—assuming there has been laboratory confirmation of their seronegative status—to maintain absolute sexual monogamy. Good intentions will not suffice. Unwavering adherence to a code of honor and trust is necessary— including the uncomfortable but requisite step of notifying one's partner immediately if there has been any extrarelationship sexual activity, and abstaining from sex with that partner until such time as testing certifies that no infection has occurred.

FEAR OF TESTING

One of the disconcerting problems in combating the spread of the AIDS virus is that many people who know they have been exposed to infection refuse to be tested to determine their antibody status. For instance, when the U.S. Centers for Disease Control conducted a national survey of the sex partners of hemophiliacs, they found that only one-third had undergone such testing.[8] This situation is particularly worrisome since it shows in a rather explicit way that education and counseling efforts with this population have been far less effective than experts had hoped. And because people need to know their HIV status so they can avoid transmitting the virus to their sex partners or, in the case of women, to their babies, this is not just an academic issue.

We have encountered a similar reluctance to be tested among the sex partners of HIV-infected drug addicts. In attempting to gather data on the rate of transmission of HIV infection from an infected man to his sex partner (correlated with the frequency and types of sexual activity engaged in by the couple), we found that the majority of women we interviewed refused to be tested. The most common reason for avoiding the test was fear: fear of finding out they might be infected, fear of being told not to become pregnant, and fear of losing their partner. Intriguingly, many of these women were resigned to the probability that they were already infected but felt that by not being tested they didn't have to confront the issue psychologically. Some of them, in fact, felt that as long as the infection wasn't "proven" scientifically, it would remain dormant. To this group, one of the primary risks of being tested was that confirmation of HIV infection would make the condition more serious, somehow activating the virus in their bodies by providing sure knowledge of its presence.

The same type of fear operates in the broader population of those who know or suspect that they have been exposed to the AIDS virus. For example, in our study group of 400 men and women with large numbers of sex partners in the preceding five years, only 3 of the 45 people who thought they were at risk had previously undergone testing on their own. Conversely, the experience at a number of public testing programs, such as those in New York City, has been that many people who are not particularly at risk for the infection rush in to be tested.

People who consider themselves at risk for HIV infection often avoid testing because they feel that finding out they are infected won't be helpful. After all, many of them point out, there is no treatment available to eradicate the infection or even to slow its progression. Furthermore, they say, discovering you're infected will only complicate your life and cause a good deal of psychological anguish as well. This sort of resignation to fate presents one of the central public health problems of the AIDS epidemic. The hundreds of thousands of carriers of the virus who go on with life as usual, oblivious to the possibility of being infected, constitute a major vector in the continuing spread of the epidemic. They are not just numbers in an epidemiological maze: they are men and women who continue to lead sexually active lives, many of them exposing multiple partners to the AIDS virus each year. They are people who, irresponsibly clinging to their personal excuses for not being tested, silently spread slow death to those with whom they couple in erotic abandon.

THE TROUBLE WITH CONDOMS

As part of the effort to combat the spread of AIDS, various experts and groups, including the U.S. Surgeon General, have strongly endorsed the use of condoms. In keeping with this recommendation, condoms have been distributed to homosexual men, on college campuses, and in other settings as part of "safe sex" kits, and a number of public education campaigns have also proclaimed that using a condom constitutes "safe sex." While it is true that condom use can effectively *reduce* the risks of unsafe sex, it is emphatically not true that condoms provide a foolproof means of avoiding exposure to the AIDS virus. Condoms can make for *safer* sex but do not guarantee safe sex.

The basic premise that a condom provides an effective mechanical barrier to the spread of the AIDS virus via semen or vaginal secretions is supported scientifically by several laboratory studies. The most relevant report involved tests of both latex and natural condoms. The condoms were filled with a fluid containing very high concentrations of the AIDS virus—about 5,000 times greater than the amounts found in semen—and were subjected to pressure, but there was no evidence that the

virus leaked out of any of the condoms tested.[9] Studies
of the same type had previously shown that viruses similar in size to the AIDS virus, such as the herpes simplex
virus, do not pass through condoms either.[10] There is
some uncertainty, however, as to whether condoms
made of natural materials such as lamb's intestine are as
effective in this regard as latex condoms.[11] This point
has not been discussed adequately in the media or in
most educational materials intended for the general public, so consumers are somewhat undereducated on this
matter. At present, at least, a cautious view suggests that
all condoms are not created equal.

Unfortunately, condoms have never been known to be
foolproof. As most people realize, they provide only a
flimsy barrier, and they are subject to manufacturing or
packaging defects that may cause them to leak. The
scope of this problem is greater than most condom users
probably realize. For example, in the spring of 1987 the
U.S. Food and Drug Administration conducted detailed
studies of the effectiveness of 204 sample lots of latex
condoms.[12] About 1 out of every 5 sample batches
leaked. While the failure rate was highest among imported brands (30 of the 98 imported sample lots failed,
compared to "only" 11 failures in the 106 domestically
manufactured sample batches), such data show that defective condoms are far from rare. Besides defects that
can occur in the manufacturing or packaging of condoms, the material the condom is made from can become
brittle as it ages or dries out.[13] Nevertheless, most
brands of condoms don't have effective storage and use
dates stamped on their packages (as is mandatory for
spermicidal creams and jellies, as well as most medica-

tions), so consumers have no way of knowing how long a batch of condoms has been on the shelf. In addition, it is obvious that condoms can be torn or punctured during use. There are no precise statistics on the frequency of this problem, but it doesn't stretch the imagination very much to see how a fingernail can tear a condom while it is being put on.

Actual use statistics—compiled not in artificial laboratory studies but in field trials by humans—rather consistently show that condoms are far from 100% effective. Most reports we have seen indicate failure rates of 10% to 15% for condoms as birth control devices.[14] While it is true that inconsistent or improper use of condoms (technically known as user failure) may be more of a problem than leaks in the condom (method failure), it is also pertinent to note that pregnancies don't occur every time a condom "fails." If we assume that pregnancy is only likely to occur during one week out of each menstrual cycle, and that a single act of unprotected intercourse during this fertile period only results in conception approximately 1 out of 8 times, the probability of pregnancy occurring from a single random failure of condom use is about 3% (that is, about 1 in 32). This means that a 10% to 15% failure rate (in terms of pregnancies) among couples using condoms consistently on each and every sexual contact during the year probably indicates an actual failure rate (in terms of "leaks") three to five times higher.

Two recent studies provide evidence that this is not just a theoretical problem. In one, Padian and her co-workers studied 97 female partners of 93 men infected with the AIDS virus.[15] They found that 23% of the

115

women were infected, and concluded, "Condom use was not significantly associated with protection from infection." In another study evaluating a group of AIDS patients and their spouses, it was found that 3 out of 18 who used condoms regularly became infected—a failure rate of 16.7%.[16]

One other aspect of condom use should be mentioned. Although a condom without leaks may provide an effective mechanical barrier to the AIDS virus contained in semen (and will also protect the penis from virus particles in vaginal or cervical secretions), unless the condom is put on virtually at the beginning of a firm erection, there is a possibility that the male's sex partner will be exposed to preejaculatory fluid containing virus.[17] Furthermore, unless the condom is removed soon after ejaculation occurs, there is a chance that semen will spill out of the condom onto the labia of the vagina or even into the vagina itself as the male's erection recedes and the condom no longer fits so tightly around the penis. Since many couples find the post-orgasmic glow a time of tenderness in which they want to lie quietly together with their genitals still in union, they run a distinct risk of having just such spillage occur. Finally, unless the penis is carefully washed to get rid of the residue of semen once a condom is removed, there may be live virus present on both the shaft and head of the penis that can certainly be contagious if rubbed against a cut or scratch or rash or blister—in fact, any abradement of the skin.

This is not to say that using condoms to reduce the risk of exposure to the AIDS virus is pointless. A good case can be made that consistent condom use will in fact provide a certain degree of protection. But to think that condom use is perfect, or even near perfect, in eliminating the risk of HIV transmission is foolishness of the highest order. Yet many medical experts, public health officials, and educators have jumped on the bandwagon proclaiming condoms are "lifesaving" devices, giving the public the impression that using condoms is all that has to be done. Though this is understandable—endorsing condom use is better than taking no action at all, and for professionals committed to dealing with the public health impact of AIDS one of the major frustrations has been how very little they've been able to recommend to a concerned public short of abstinence from sex and illicit drugs—to suggest that condom use is a complete answer in the fight against AIDS is to oversimplify and mislead in an irresponsible fashion.

MAKING UNSAFE SEX SAFER

For those whose partners are unwilling to undergo voluntary testing in order to establish that they're free of infection with the AIDS virus, virtually any sex act carries with it a certain degree of risk. Even as seemingly innocuous an act as mutual manual stimulation of the genitals is not completely risk-free. If preejaculatory fluid or semen comes in contact with a sore, a cut, or a rash on the partner's hand or body, there is a possibility of infection. Likewise, if a man stimulating his partner's genitals inserts a finger into her vagina, he will come in skin contact with vaginal secretions that may be infected. If

117

there is a break in the skin of his finger or hand, or if he subsequently touches another part of his body where there is a break in the skin, he runs a small but distinct risk of infection.

One possible solution to this quandary would be for sex partners of uncertain testing status to wear disposable plastic gloves during all intimate moments. These gloves, after all, aren't too different from condoms. Yet we are unwilling to seriously entertain such an outlandish notion—right now, it seems so unnatural and artificial as to violate the essential dignity of humanity. A better (that is, less offensive-sounding) solution might be for partners to use nonoxynol-9-containing creams or jellies for genital stimulatory activities, since it has been shown that nonoxynol-9, which is the active chemical ingredient in a number of spermicides, effectively kills the AIDS virus.[18]

Couples with unknown HIV status, or couples in which one partner is known to be infected, should absolutely avoid anal intercourse. Based on present evidence, there seems to be little doubt that anal intercourse is the riskiest form of sexual activity. To engage in anal coitus when there is a possibility that one partner is infected is to tempt fate—and biological reality—too strongly. In our judgment, relying on condom use for anal intercourse when one partner is infected or when one or both partners have unknown HIV status is still taking an unwarranted risk that is compounded over time if the activity is repeated.

Similarly, if we are to give credence to the data from Africa and to our own findings, it is unacceptably risky to engage in penile-vaginal intercourse when one or both partners' HIV status is unknown or when one partner is known to be infected. In the absence of studies showing that this risk is significantly reduced by the use of condoms, to rely on condoms for truly safe sex—or even a reasonable approximation of safe sex—is to blatantly disregard the facts. The condom industry, of course, will take grave exception to this statement. Readers can expect a rather vitriolic critique of our recommendations about condoms from this group, which has a vested economic interest in maintaining the illusion that condoms confer an adequate degree of protection against the AIDS virus.

Oral-genital sex presents a somewhat different problem. Here, at least as of late 1987, there is a lack of substantive research documenting the relative degree of risk associated with oral sex by itself. In one study of homosexual men in San Francisco, there did not seem to be any statistically significant increased risk of HIV infection among men who engaged in oral-genital sex compared to those who didn't—although 24% of the men who had any history of oral-genital contact were infected, compared to 18.2% of those who had not engaged in oral-genital sex.[19] As we pointed out in Chapter 2, this study did not make any attempt to quantify the frequency or number of oral-genital contacts, so that a man who reported performing fellatio once in the two years preceding the study was placed in the same group, for statistical purposes, as a man who performed fellatio dozens of times a month. This may explain why these researchers found no indication that oral-genital sex was associated with an increased risk of infection with the AIDS virus. However, in a study of 45 adults with AIDS and their spouses, 12 of 26 spouses who participated in repeated oral sex became infected during the study, whereas only 2 out of 19 uninfected spouses regularly engaged in oral sex.[20]

In light of this uncertainty, until more definitive evidence is available, oral-genital sex should be avoided unless it is known that both partners are HIV-free. Using a condom while performing fellatio is not only aesthetically distasteful to most people, it also increases the likelihood of the condom's being torn by contact with teeth—a mechanical hazard that condoms were not manufactured to endure.

We should also add that any type of sexual activity posing a significant risk of exposure to a partner's blood should particularly be avoided when both partners are not known to be free of HIV infection. In this category we include not only the obvious, such as sadomasochistic sex that involves beatings, whipping, or the use of needles, pins, or other sharp objects, but also vigorous biting or scratching or any kind of sex play that can cause bleeding, since blood can certainly transmit the AIDS virus via nongenital erotic contact. In addition, although no reliable research has yet been done on this topic, it is probably wise to avoid coitus, cunnilingus, or finger insertion into the vagina during a woman's menstrual flow if her HIV status is uncertain.

In short, this is a time for considerable caution in sexual conduct. The need for caution is most pronounced in terms of choosing a partner. Prostitutes, male homosexuals, IV drug abusers, males with bisexual experiences, and people who have had large numbers of sexual partners are especially risky as sex partners until it can be shown by testing that they are free of HIV infection. Trusting attitudes should be tempered by the seriousness of the current situation: since you can't tell if people are infected with the AIDS virus by how they look, and since you can't really rely on their own recitation of their sexual history, you are just being prudent by insisting that someone who wants to get in bed with you accompany you to a clinic for testing first.

8

BEYOND THE
SEXUAL REVOLUTION

If the 1960s and 1970s were a time of freewheeling sexual experimentation, one-night stands, and instant gratification, have the late 1980s become an era of sexual fear and inhibition as a direct result of the onslaught of widely publicized epidemics of sexually transmitted diseases such as genital herpes and AIDS? To examine this question, we will first consider the changes that have already occurred in gay male patterns of sexual behavior in large metropolitan areas where the message about AIDS has been delivered most intensively. Next we will look at current trends in sexual behavior among young adults, since this segment of the population has often served as a harbinger of change in the broader population. Finally we will discuss the sexual impact of the AIDS epidemic on adolescents.

SEXUAL BEHAVIOR CHANGES
IN GAY MEN

Judging from newspaper accounts and the somewhat self-congratulatory statements of community leaders, educators, and others, it would appear that gay men have rather universally adopted "safer sex" practices and are now dealing so effectively with the issue of sexual transmission of AIDS that new infections have dropped off considerably in number. Various experts cite data showing a decrease in cases of rectal gonorrhea[1] and a reduction in the number of sex partners among male homosexuals[2] as proof of such changes. Unfortunately, a closer look at sexual practices among gay (and bisexual) men today gives a less optimistic picture of the terrain.*

We can get a first approximation of what is happening by looking at the behavior of a group of carefully selected homosexual men in New York City and Washington, D.C. Homosexuals in these two cities, needless to say, have been the target audience of massive educational campaigns led by gays themselves, public health

---

*Even if gay males change their sexual behavior, it must be asked whether the changes are substantive enough to lessen their risk of acquiring AIDS. This requires looking at behavioral changes in relation to the prevalence of HIV infection within the population in question. For example, if the prevalence of HIV infection in gay men in San Francisco increased from 50% to 75% over a three-year period, then a 20% or 30% reduction in risky sexual practices wouldn't compensate for the increased risk of infection because of the higher prevalence.

experts, community leaders, and legislators. The message they've been getting boils down to several essential points, perhaps the strongest of which is the great riskiness inherent in anal sex. But in 1986, according to Dr. James J. Goedert of the National Cancer Institute—one of this country's leading workers in the field of AIDS—48% of this group of "highly educated and motivated" homosexual men continued to have anal intercourse, and 77% of those who practiced anal sex did not use condoms.[3]

It is also instructive to look at data from San Francisco, where the gay community is probably more organized and politically cohesive than elsewhere in the United States. Early intensive educational campaigns aimed at promoting behavioral change among gay men there have been frequently cited as successful, yet a major research report from San Francisco found that in a sample of 796 homosexual or bisexual men studied from June 1984 to January 1985, 312 reported having 10 to 49 male sex partners in the two previous years, while 195—almost a quarter of the sample—reported having at least 50 male sex partners during this time.[4] Furthermore, among 729 men for whom data were reported, only 99 abstained from anal intercourse. It is difficult to call this evidence of considerable sexual restraint.

Because San Francisco may be a somewhat atypical area in regard to sexual behavior patterns of homosexual men, it is useful to consider what is happening in other parts of the country. In 1987 we surveyed a group of 200 homosexual men in metropolitan areas in the northeastern United States, using a self-administered questionnaire to determine how their sexual behavior patterns had changed as a result of concern about the AIDS epidemic.[5] We expected to find a dramatic drop in the annual number of sex partners these men had over the five-year period between 1982 and 1986. The data (Table 8.1) were somewhat surprising to us, since there was much less of a decline in the current number of sex partners than we had anticipated. In fact, more than 20% of the men we surveyed had actually increased their number of sex partners, seemingly in disregard of the AIDS epidemic raging around them. It should also be noted that even with the reduction in annual number of sex partners reported by the majority, they averaged 26.9 partners per person.

Of the 172 men in our sample who reported having engaged in anal sex during 1981 and 1982, 101 continued this practice during 1986 and 1987 (see Table 8.2). Remarkably—and closely supporting the data reported by Goedert—75 of these 101 men who continued

---

TABLE 8.1
Annual Number of Homosexual Partners for a Cohort of 200
Homosexual Men Ages 21-35, Northeastern United States

	DISTRIBUTION OF COHORT BY YEAR									
	1982		1983		1984		1985		1986	
# OF PARTNERS	#	%	#	%	#	%	#	%	#	%
None	4	2.0	4	2.0	5	2.5	4	2.0	6	3.0
One	16	8.0	15	7.5	16	8.0	19	9.5	20	10.0
2–5	21	10.5	23	11.5	22	11.0	28	14.0	31	15.5
6–9	18	9.0	19	9.5	24	12.0	23	11.5	29	14.5
10–24	41	20.5	40	20.0	37	18.5	33	16.5	27	13.5
24–49	52	26.0	51	25.5	52	26.0	51	25.5	48	24.0
≥ 50	48	24.0	48	24.0	44	22.0	42	21.0	39	19.5

TABLE 8.2

Self-Reported Participation in Anal Intercourse for a Cohort of 200 Homosexual Men Ages 21–35, Northeastern United States

	YEAR	
	1981–82	1986–87
Engaged in		
Anal Intercourse		
Yes	172 (86%)	101 (50.5%)
No	28 (14%)	99 (49.5%)
Condom Use During		
Anal Intercourse[a]		
Always	—	12/101
Regularly	—	14/101
Sometimes	—	18/101
Infrequently	—	34/101
Never	—	23/101

[a]The frequency categories were defined as follows: Always = 100% of the time; Regularly = at least 75% of the time but less than 100%; Sometimes = at least 25% of the time but less than 75%; Infrequently = at least once, but less than 25% of the time. It should be noted that in 1981–82 virtually no homosexual men were using condoms since it had not yet been determined that AIDS is a sexually transmitted disease.

anal intercourse did not use condoms regularly, despite extensive educational campaigns geared at eliminating anal sex without use of condoms. Another point repetitively and loudly made to the gay male community is that anonymous sex can be lethal in the era of AIDS. The message is—quite correctly—be selective and know your partners. However, 62% of the 200 men in the overall homosexual sample reported that more than half of their sex partners were strangers. These numbers are a harsh reminder that patterns of human sexual behavior are not

as easily amenable to change as might be imagined—
especially considering that almost every man in our survey knew at least one person who had died of AIDS.

Here are some of the comments these men made in
explaining why they continued to engage in what must
certainly be considered high-risk activities:

A 32-year-old hair stylist: For all the know-it-alls, moralists,
and experts, let me say this: I'd rather be dead than be
celibate.

A 29-year-old stockbroker: We all take risks every day of our
lives. Riding the subway or crossing the street is risky.
Without sex and without excitement, life wouldn't be
much worth living to me.

A 35-year-old physician: There's a fair amount of denial
going on, as there is with any self-destructive behavior.
But some of us are hooked on sex just as strongly—or
maybe more strongly—as an alcoholic needs his bottle or
an addict needs his fix. I only wish this epidemic had
started with heterosexuals. What sort of advice about
abstinence would have been given then?

A 26-year-old electrician: The way I look at it is this. Ciga-
rettes will kill me if I don't stop smoking. I'll get cirrhosis
if I drink too much. If I do crack, I may have a heart
attack. Or maybe some crazy politician will start a nuclear
war and we'll all be dead. Personally, I don't plan to slow
down my sex life just because someone tells me I could
get sick.

Embodied in such responses are various themes we've
heard over and over again, not just from gay males but
from many heterosexuals too. There is a strong degree
of fatalism or determinism. "Chances are I've already

127

been exposed." "If it's going to happen, it's going to happen." There is rejection of the reality of the risk. "We all take risks all the time." "AIDS isn't as much of a problem here as it is in New York City or San Francisco." There is denial that it could happen "to me." There is resistance against being told what to do. There is a very legitimate wish to be autonomous and self-actualizing. Among gay men there is a belief that one shouldn't repudiate one's sexual identity by abstinence from homosexual acts. And there is an implicit rejection of the idea that two men should form a monogamous sexual relationship for the sole purpose of hiding from the ravages of an epidemic disease, even while there is acceptance of those who choose this path as a survival mechanism, a sort of compromise between their sexual impulses and their sense of self-preservation.

None of this is to say that there is no fear in the gay male community, because fear of AIDS is almost palpable. Cavalier attitudes may mask the fear much of the time, but fear also contributes to a sense of excitement in what is dangerous and forbidden. Fear surfaces for some of these men when they wonder whether the anonymous partner of the night before might have been infected with the AIDS virus. Fear breaks through when a rash or pimple appears on the skin and the thought "My God, it's Kaposi's sarcoma" scampers through the mind, only to be quickly brushed aside with an attitude not too different from that of second-year medical students who worry about being afflicted with almost every disease they study. Fear comes home to roost most strongly, perhaps, when a man learns that one of his sex partners has been diagnosed as having AIDS. Yet even this news—a thunderbolt of reality—does not motivate most homosexual men to abstain completely from risky sexual practices. In fact, this amalgamation of fears seems to drive some—including some who know they are infected[6]—to almost manic bouts of sexual activity.

Here is one of the clear problems of the AIDS epidemic. Many gay men who know they are infected with the AIDS virus are continuing to have sex with other men. In fact, even some men who have been diagnosed as having full-blown AIDS have continued to have sex with numerous partners. Though leaders of the gay community are aware of such practices—which might easily be seen as homophobic acts—they have not spoken out in strong language to get across the message that such irresponsible behavior is extraordinarily destructive to the gay community and the gay cause. But as one gay activist remarked, "If we all get AIDS and die, we've just managed to prove that Jerry Falwell's a prophet."[7]

We do not mean to say that homosexuals are more compulsive about sex than heterosexuals or less responsible in following rational public health guidelines aimed at reducing the risks of continuing sexual transmission of AIDS. Many gay men have drastically changed their sexual behavior; some practice what they feel (or have been told) is "safe sex" virtually all the time, and others have formed one-to-one monogamous relationships to weather the storm. Instead, what we are saying is that heterosexuals and homosexuals are apt to be very much alike—which means that producing broad enough changes in everyone's sexual behavior will require a much more extensive, inventive, and multidimensional campaign than has yet been seen.

THE IMPACT OF AIDS
ON HETEROSEXUAL BEHAVIOR

There has been a curious dichotomy in the response of heterosexuals to the AIDS epidemic. While many heterosexuals voice concern about AIDS and a few are so frightened that their response borders on phobia, it seems to be mainly the same group of highly educated, upper-middle-class whites who were cautious sexually during the genital herpes scare of 1979–1982 who are being cautious today. Most heterosexuals, especially those who are poorer and less educated, still regard the AIDS epidemic as far removed from their lives; they see it as a disease affecting homosexuals, bisexuals, and drug addicts, rather than a disease with direct personal relevance. (The one notable exception is that according to several public opinion polls, the majority of heterosexuals seem to be worried about the possibility of being infected with the AIDS virus through a tainted blood transfusion.)

As we reported in Chapter 4, the segment of the heterosexual population that is most sexually active in terms of number of partners hasn't let fear of AIDS alter their behavior very substantially. These persons continue to have multiple sex partners without making much of an attempt to use condoms regularly. Furthermore, there has been no noticeable drop in their participation in anal intercourse, despite particular emphasis in the media on the fact that this is a high-risk form of sexual activity. However, since this group, which is clearly a

distinct minority of the broader heterosexual population, may be the most resistant to change, it is instructive
to see what is happening in other populations of heterosexuals at present.

Dr. Sheldon H. Landesman, who heads the AIDS
study group at the State University of New York Health
Science Center in Brooklyn, estimated that in mid-1987
there were 15,000 to 20,000 women in New York City
alone who had been infected with the AIDS virus because their sex partners had used contaminated needles.[8] Other experts say that at least 50,000 women in
New York City—3% of the women of reproductive age—
are asymptomatic carriers of HIV.[9] Black and Hispanic
women have been particularly hard hit: for these minority groups, "the cumulative incidence rates for AIDS [the
disease] acquired by heterosexual contact with an intravenous drug abuser were more than 24 times those for
white women."[10] And though it seems that inner city
women are well educated about risk factors for infection
with the AIDS virus, relatively few are modifying their
behavior as a result.[11] A number of researchers have
reported that most women who know they are in high-
risk groups do not insist that their partners use condoms.
Even among women who know they are infected and
realize they can pass the infection to their sex partners,
condom use is haphazard at best.

Another perspective on the heterosexual scene comes
from scrutinizing an aspect of sexual behavior that—
aside from *Mayflower Madam*—seems to have been nearly
forgotten in the midst of the sexual revolution. But the
profession of prostitution has not only endured, it has
become one of the principal vectors in spreading the

AIDS virus to the heterosexual world. Consider these statistics compiled in a six-city study by the Centers for Disease Control:[12]

- In Las Vegas 26% of prostitutes tested were infected with the AIDS virus.
- In Colorado Springs 27% were infected.
- In San Francisco 74 out of 157 prostitutes (47%) were infected.
- Even higher rates of infection were found in Miami (180 out of 309, or 58%), in Los Angeles (152 out of 217, or 70%), and in Newark (51 out of 59, or 86%).

The client population being served by these women includes men from virtually all walks of life; salesmen, accountants, lawyers, doctors, gas station attendants, servicemen, and others are all being exposed to the AIDS virus as a result of visits to prostitutes. Though there is probably a far greater chance of becoming infected from sexual contact with a streetwalker than with a high-priced call girl, prostitutes at any price level who know they are carrying the virus do not instantly stop working as a public service gesture. One has to wonder why men would be so foolish as to risk exposure to the AIDS virus by patronizing a prostitute, but someone is out there keeping the nation's tens of thousands of prostitutes employed. This, too, will inevitably lead to an explosive upsurge in the rate of heterosexual infection with the AIDS virus.

In 1986 we conducted a survey of a heterosexual population distinctly different from the inner city women and prostitutes referred to above. Our sample consisted of 425 single heterosexual adults (210 males and 215 females) in New York, St. Louis, and Los Angeles.[13] All were in their twenties, 94% were white, and two-thirds had at least one year of college education, although none were full-time students at the time of the study. In this population 72% of the women and 63% of the men said they had become more cautious about sex as a result of worries about AIDS, but many respondents did not seem to have translated this concern into consistent behavioral change. For example, 47% of the women didn't insist that their partners use condoms, and 64% of them indicated that they had had unprotected intercourse at least "a few times" in the preceding year; 76% of the men indicated that they did not use condoms on a regular basis.

Nevertheless, this group of single young adults did show some evidence of caution in regard to AIDS: 79% of the women and 74% of the men said that they were more selective in deciding with whom and when they would have sex. This reported change of attitude seems to be borne out by one interesting finding: both men and women reported a small but significant reduction in number of sex partners for the year immediately preceding the survey compared to the previous year. For men, the mean number of partners decreased from 3.8 to 2.5, and for women, from 2.6 to 1.9. While it cannot be shown conclusively that the decrease resulted from caution directly related to the AIDS epidemic, our intuitive interpretation of the data is that this was the case. Our viewpoint is buttressed by comments such as these from the young adult sample:

A 24-year-old man: When I read all this stuff about AIDS, it looks pretty bad. You can't tell who's got it and who hasn't. So instead of being a playboy, I'm living with someone now. It's not so bad either.

A 27-year-old divorced woman: Before I got married, I used to be pretty wild. Now I'm too scared by all the statistics about AIDS. How am I going to know that a guy I meet in a bar isn't bisexual? Why take that kind of risk or have that sort of worry?

A 25-year-old man: I heard on TV that now when you sleep with someone, you're really sleeping with everyone else they've had sex with in the last ten years. That shook me up. So I'm very choosy now, very much more a one-woman man.

On the other hand, there was no uniformity of opinion in this group. About a quarter of the respondents felt that they had no risk of being sexually exposed to AIDS. An even larger number felt confident that AIDS is primarily confined to gays, bisexuals, and addicts, and that if they guarded against contact with those persons, they would have essentially no exposure to AIDS in the everyday heterosexual world. Alarmingly, more than 1 out of 8 young adults in our survey didn't realize that AIDS could be transmitted sexually from a woman to a man. Also of interest was the finding that of the 53% of women who insisted on condom use, more than a quarter gave in when their partners objected or refused. Apparently, many young single women are not so clearly convinced that the risk of HIV transmission applies to them that they will refuse to participate in sex if the male won't use a condom.

Many heterosexual men—especially but not exclusively those who are less well educated—scoff at the idea of using a condom. They see the condom as a nuisance, a barrier to physical pleasure, and a sign of weakness: the condom is symbolic both of giving in to the wishes of a female partner, which threatens their sense of virility, and of acknowledging that it is legitimate to be afraid of the AIDS virus, which is also threatening. More sophisticated, better-educated heterosexual men often object to using condoms on the very scientific grounds we've raised—that condoms are imperfect. These men are more apt to acquiesce to using condoms—at least for a while—because they understand that it may be their ticket to sexual access. Most of them know from prior experience that once they've established an ongoing sexual relationship in which a woman feels that she's getting to know the man, it will probably be easy to agree on discarding condoms entirely.

Though many heterosexual adults have adopted an attitude of sexual caution, there is still a sizable group for whom one-night stands and freewheeling sex go on much as in the 1970s. Singles bars continue to thrive in most cities; newspaper and magazine classified personal ads continue to unite lonely partners; and even swingers clubs, complete with organized picnics, mate swapping, and occasional group sex, still hold some allure for thousands of participants. This is a segment of the heterosexual world that has not been systematically studied. However, if our research on heterosexuals who have numerous sex partners is applicable here, as we assume it to be, then this is the volcanic underside of the AIDS epidemic—and in a short while it will erupt.

At the other extreme is a small category of heterosexuals who can best be classified as phobic about the possibility of becoming infected with the AIDS virus. (Phobias about what used to be called "venereal disease" are not new by any means.[14]) The phobia can range from avid avoidance of all sexual situations to more extreme manifestations. In one case a 33-year-old single woman keeps a scrapbook of news clippings about AIDS, with the first page showing a neatly colored bar chart on which she records the periodic death count released by the CDC. In another version of this phobia a 40-year-old man wears surgeon's gloves whenever he goes shopping in Manhattan, and refuses to shake hands with anyone. In still another case a previously healthy woman insists she's been exposed to the virus by her ex-boyfriend and goes to several different doctors each month requesting a blood test to find out if she's infected. Of course, these phobic reactions are nothing to joke about. They show how fear, uncertainty, and a sense of our own mortality can coalesce to cause severe emotional anguish when we are faced with a crisis that we seem to be helpless to control.

ADOLESCENTS AND AIDS

Thus far AIDS has primarily affected adults in the 20-to-40-year age bracket, but experts fear that teenagers will be the next major target of the epidemic. Many teens are sexually active, and many teens use drugs; both activities put them right in the path of a speeding locomotive.

The best statistics on teenage sexual activity come from studies done at the Johns Hopkins University School of Public Health.[15] According to these reports, 60% to 70% of older unmarried teenage females have coital experience; even among 15-year-olds, more than 1 in 5 are sexually active. Among black teenage females the numbers are even more striking: 75% of 17-year-olds and 89% of unmarried 19-year-olds are not virgins. Beyond these statistics, one other important reality of teenage sex should be mentioned: there are more than a million pregnancies among American teenagers every year.[16]

It is clear that there was a major change in sexual behavior in America in the late 1960s and 1970s, one of the most notable trends being that teenage females became sexually active at younger and younger ages.[17] Although there is some preliminary evidence that this trend may have leveled off by 1982,[18] there does not appear to be any indication that either the genital herpes scare, a swing to political conservatism, or the current AIDS epidemic has convinced most teenagers that abstinence is the wisest course. Campaigns that urge teenagers to "just say NO"—a slogan used in reference to both sex and drugs—do not seem to have worked very well so far.

Teenage patterns of illicit drug use have also shown recent evidence of leveling off or even declining slightly since the late 1970s and early 1980s.[19] Nevertheless, there are millions of teenagers experimenting with drugs, and an estimated 500,000 who inject drugs,[20] thus placing themselves at risk of acquiring the AIDS virus by using contaminated needles and syringes. In addition, it is thought that over 100,000 teenagers, both female and male, become involved in prostitution each year,[21] which also puts them at high risk for infection.

American adolescents as a group are notoriously irresponsible about their sexual activity, as shown by the extremely high rate of unintended teenage pregnancy (the highest in the Western hemisphere[22]) and by extraordinarily high rates of infection with sexually transmitted diseases.[23] Most American teenagers don't use contraception; most of those who do use it haphazardly at best.[24] Teenage males are especially unwilling to use condoms, often considering it unmanly, unnatural, inconvenient, and unnecessary.[25] No wonder, then, that adolescents seem to be particularly vulnerable to infection with the AIDS virus.

So far, at least, school-based education about AIDS has been too little, too timid, and too unrealistic to accurately inform our teenagers or to convince them that AIDS is not just another threat invented by adults to curtail their independence and fun. Many of the curricula supposedly teaching teens about the AIDS epidemic don't discuss homosexuality or bisexuality at all; others don't mention condoms; still others give the message that abstinence is the only way to avoid a terrible death. The inadequacies of school-based education about AIDS can be seen in the findings of a 1986 survey of over 800 Massachusetts teenagers 16 to 19 years old.[26] More than half of these adolescents erroneously believed that infection with the AIDS virus can result from donating blood, and 29% did not know that the virus can be passed from females to males. Most said that they were not worried about getting AIDS, which was reflected in another alarming statistic: although 70% said they were sexually active, only 15% had made any changes in their sexual behavior because of concern about AIDS. Of those who were concerned and attempted to change their sexual behavior, only 1 in 5 did so in a way that could be judged effective.

The findings of a 1987 survey involving more than 350 college students at Syracuse University do not present a more optimistic scenario.[27] For instance, most of the students interviewed showed a "great lack of knowledge and factual data about AIDS" and felt that they had little or no risk of exposure to AIDS since they were not in high-risk groups. As the authors of this study noted, "Often unconcerned about risk, they failed to see that high risk *behaviors* placed them in jeopardy." Not only did the students show a high level of denial, most of them mistakenly thought that they could intuitively know or sense which of their potential sex partners were safe and which weren't. In addition, although college students might be thought to have fewer hang-ups about sex than older people, these students weren't comfortable with the idea of talking about AIDS or condoms with their sexual partners, and many said that they did not use condoms at all. "In general," the authors noted, "students equated 'safer sex' with 'not-for-fun' sex."

Here are comments from several high school and college students that show the range of teenage attitudes about AIDS:

A 17-year-old boy: Everyone knows that AIDS isn't a problem if you're not gay and you don't shoot up.

139

A 15-year-old girl: My mother says that you can get AIDS from shaking hands with someone who's got it, but I don't think that's true. But I worry that I could get it from having sex with someone.

A 16-year-old girl: There's no way I could catch AIDS, because my boyfriend doesn't do drugs. Anyway, I heard you only catch it if you have sex during your period.

An 18-year-old boy: I heard on TV that you can only get AIDS from having sex with men.

A 19-year-old girl: I don't think I need to be worried about AIDS at all. I don't jump into bed with just anyone I meet, and I wouldn't sleep with a guy who looks like he's been using drugs. [This teenager had had seven different sex partners in the preceding year.]

A 17-year-old boy: From what I can see, all this fuss about AIDS is pretty much exaggerated. I mean, it's a problem if you use dirty needles or if you are bisexual or gay, but I've only slept with three girls this year, and I knew them all pretty well.

A 16-year-old girl: AIDS is pretty scary to me. I'm still a virgin, and I plan to keep it that way for a while. What's the point in taking a chance with your life?

Just as some teenagers believe that you can't get pregnant if you have sex standing up or that you can't contract a sexually transmitted disease from someone you love, many teens have taken a stance toward AIDS that is based on wishful but woefully misinformed thinking. A sex education teacher told us, for example, about a high school student who was certain that the AIDS virus is only transmitted heterosexually by pregnant women.

Another student was convinced that the virus is only contracted by those who engage in anal sex. When such serious misconceptions are added to the ordinary difficulties of adolescence, the tendency to wait for a crisis rather than thinking in terms of prevention, and the strong sense most teens have of their own invulnerability, it is no wonder that they have scarcely retreated—if at all—from the recent sexual revolution.

IS THE SEXUAL REVOLUTION OVER?

While it seems fairly clear to us that the sexual revolution is no longer careening along on its carefree course, what we have actually seen in the broad population is a leveling off in the rate of sexual experimentation rather than a reversion to the values of earlier days. Premarital sex is not frowned on today as it was in the 1950s;[28] extramarital sex has not disappeared overnight; young adults are not hooking up in exclusively monogamous relationships with much sense of urgency. Unless adolescents and young adults can be convinced that the AIDS virus is a reality in their world right now, it is unlikely that there will be enough of a shift in behavior to keep this epidemic from expanding at an alarming rate. Although it makes a nice headline, the sexual revolution is not yet dead—it's just that some of the troops are dying.

9

AIDS PREVENTION
AS AN ISSUE FOR SOCIETY

America is now in a difficult position in regard to the
AIDS epidemic. No cohesive national policy has been
devised to deal with issues of prevention. No carefully
planned, priority-ranked research agenda has been
mapped out and agreed upon. There has been much too
little economic planning for patient care and other costs
that will be associated with the epidemic over the next
decade. And there is considerable disagreement over
how to protect the civil rights of people with AIDS, people infected with the AIDS virus, and uninfected people
in high-risk groups while at the same time fulfilling another legitimate function of government—protecting
public health.

It's easy to be a civil libertarian when gonorrhea is the
worst sexually transmitted disease raging in the land.
Penicillin works reasonably well as a cure, and gonorrhea
rarely kills people. But in the age of AIDS our society will
be faced with much more difficult choices—choices that
will descend upon us in an avalanche of painful awareness and expense in a few years unless we begin to plan
carefully and sensibly today. In this chapter we will make

a number of suggestions for dealing with these challenges.

EDUCATION

There is little question that an intensive, comprehensive educational campaign must be a primary component of any effort to control the spread of HIV infection. Such a campaign will only be effective, however, if it does more than disseminate facts: unless education results in concrete changes in sexual behavior and a meaningful reduction in the sharing of contaminated needles and syringes, it is unlikely to serve a useful public health function. To produce these sorts of changes, education must motivate as well as inform.

Unfortunately, educational efforts thus far have been, as the Institute of Medicine and the National Academy of Sciences put it, "woefully inadequate."[1] To improve this situation, a number of urgent steps must be taken.

1. *A comprehensive AIDS curriculum must be developed for extensive use in public schools.* To be effective, such a program must start well before young people begin to engage in sexual activity and drug use. This means that public school education about AIDS should be implemented no later than the fourth or fifth grade.[2] While the level of sophistication will obviously deepen with older students, repeated reinforcement of the prevention message at each grade level is nec-

essary to maximize the utility of the education effort. In addition, since AIDS education requires concomitant sex and drug education, we will have to rethink the timing and content of the presentation of such subjects in an integrated manner in all public schools. Furthermore, unless such courses offer fairly explicit discussion of sexual behavior—including frank discussion of homosexuality, bisexuality, sexual intercourse, and oral and anal sex—it is unlikely that school educational efforts will do much good.

2. *Special education programs must be targeted at specific high-risk groups, including IV drug users, homosexual men, pregnant women, men who have sexual contact with prostitutes, and heterosexuals who have sex with multiple partners.* Each of these groups requires a somewhat different approach in the style, content, and emphasis of the educational effort. While the first priority in educating IV drug users may well be to strongly discourage needle sharing, it is also important to encourage this population to be voluntarily tested for HIV infection and to provide them with information regarding the risks of sexual transmission. Education aimed at pregnant women or women who are considering pregnancy must of course have a very different emphasis. Unless specific educational campaigns are tailored to the needs and demographics of target groups and delivered in a manner that reaches the intended audience, they will be unlikely to achieve anything close to maximal effectiveness.

3. *A broad-based multimedia general education campaign that models responsible behavior should be undertaken as soon as*

possible. This type of educational effort should be an ongoing one. What is needed is assistance from scriptwriters and producers who agree to incorporate warnings about the AIDS epidemic in their prime-time shows or cinematic efforts. If actors like Michael J. Fox, Tom Cruise, Debra Winger, and Molly Ringwald stopped to discuss the risk of AIDS before jumping into bed with a new sex partner or even indicated that there were legitimate health reasons for saying no to sex, a powerful message would be conveyed to the viewing public—especially teenagers and young adults. Similarly, if a saturation campaign were undertaken with magazine, radio, and television interviews (or even spot "endorsements") in which well-known athletes and other celebrities discussed the risks and realities of infection with the AIDS virus, the educational message would be received far more effectively than it has been so far.

4. *All colleges and universities should provide their students extensive educational and counseling services related to AIDS prevention.* As we have already discussed, many adolescents and young adults on college campuses around the country don't feel that they're at risk for HIV infection. Since these students are particularly likely to be experimenting with sex and drug use, it is imperative that college health services act to prevent infection, instead of just dealing with it once it has occurred. We recommend that all incoming students receive a packet of written materials about the AIDS epidemic and be required to attend, at a minimum, a two-hour seminar on AIDS prevention during the

145

first week of classes or during an orientation period before classes formally begin. Ideally, additional presentations on the topic should be made periodically throughout the academic year so the message is not entirely forgotten. We also strongly suggest that a consortium of colleges, perhaps under the auspices of an existing educational organization, undertake the preparation of a set of instructional materials, including video resources, geared to the college audience.

5. *Primary care physicians should assume an active role in educating patients about the risks of HIV infection and how to avoid exposure.* Before this can be done effectively, physicians themselves must be reasonably up-to-date on the facts about HIV transmission and testing. Unfortunately, many physicians are woefully uninformed about the AIDS epidemic—and the situation isn't likely to improve in the near future unless a federal agency such as the CDC or the Public Health Service (perhaps acting in concert with an organization like the American Medical Association) makes a concerted effort to provide thorough continuing medical education on this subject. This might be done either through the production of a set of videotapes to be distributed to all hospitals, clinics, medical schools, and office-based primary care physicians in the country, or through a multi-city satellite TV education program. Such an effort would be costly, but the result would be extraordinarily helpful in the overall prevention effort—especially since physicians are probably in the best position of all to know which

people are engaging in activities that place them at a high risk of exposure to the AIDS virus, and to offer appropriate counsel.

6. *To coordinate and implement the entire educational effort, a special office should be created in the U.S. Department of Health and Human Services, as recommended by the Institute of Medicine and the National Academy of Sciences;* [3] *this office must be given ample budgetary support and broad latitude in its mission.* Without a nationally coordinated effort, it is unlikely that education will make much of a difference in containing the spread of this epidemic. As a practical matter, such a campaign will certainly need to enlist the help of experts from advertising, the media, and the world of education. But the key to the campaign, in many ways, will be the explicitness and veracity of the preventive advice that is given. Admonitions to avoid "unsafe sex" are too vague to influence many people: it will be necessary to be more specific about just what should be done. Likewise, pretending that condoms make for "safe sex" when virtually all health experts realize that this isn't true is a highly irresponsible position for an educational campaign.

In the final analysis, while education is of considerable importance in alerting people to the realities of the AIDS epidemic and in forestalling misunderstandings and visceral reactions that lead to unwarranted discrimination against people who have AIDS, we believe that education alone will not be highly effective in preventing the continuing spread of HIV infection. In our view, unless edu-

147

cational efforts are supported by a number of other testing, counseling, and research programs, the goal of prevention will not be reached in this century.

RESEARCH

We believe that the amount of federal and state funding allocated to date for AIDS-related research has been far too little to accomplish what needs to be done. There are a number of important efforts in the biomedical area that must be promptly and intensively addressed, and there is a marked need for a central office to coordinate the overall approach. Since these points have been carefully delineated by the Institute of Medicine and the National Academy of Sciences,[4] we will not discuss them here. However, several areas of *applied* research that we see as necessary right now warrant brief mention.

- A large-scale national probability sample should be studied to ascertain better prevalence figures for HIV infection than are now available and to correlate HIV status with a detailed look at sexual behavior, drug use, and coexistent medical illnesses, particularly other sexually transmitted diseases.

- Several major projects should be undertaken to evaluate the types of educational strategies that result in the most meaningful risk-reduction behavior for various population groups, including teenagers, racial minorities, illicit drug users, bisexuals, and others.

- Prospective epidemiological studies must be started in couples for whom the onset of HIV infection can be pinpointed in one partner reasonably precisely to develop better data on the specific risks of transmission associated with particular types of sexual activity.

- Gender differences in the natural history of HIV infection, including possible differences in transmission rates and rates of progression of the infection, should be carefully examined.

SPECIAL PROGRAMS FOR DRUG ABUSE

In light of the rising rates of HIV infection among the nation's drug addicts, it is imperative to take action now to cut down on needle-sharing practices. The best way of accomplishing this, we believe, is to greatly expand the number and capacity of methadone treatment programs in urban areas. While this will require a large amount of federal, state, and city funding, failure to move quickly will only result in a dizzying escalation of costs some four or five years down the road as the number of people sick with AIDS and ARC spirals upward.

Methadone programs will not, of course, reach the entire drug-abusing population. Thus, it is also important to hire teams of former addicts—who are familiar with the lingo and problems of the drug scene, as well as the excuses drug users are apt to give—to handle outreach programs in which they teach as many drug users as possible how and why to sterilize their needles and syringes. This is certainly not a solution to the problem, but since drugs seem to be an almost permanent part of our culture at present, it is a measure that will help save lives.

CIVIL RIGHTS ISSUES

Various civil liberties organizations and gay rights groups have expressed considerable alarm over the prevailing climate of public concern about the AIDS epidemic. While we do not intend to address the broad range of these issues here—including matters as diverse (and important) as the appropriateness of deciding when, if ever, to ban infected children from public school classrooms, the ethical propriety of physicians refusing to care for patients with AIDS, or the policies employers should adopt in regard to workers who are infected with the AIDS virus—we do want to address certain aspects of the civil rights issues that are most pertinent to the social policy recommendations we will make in the remainder of this chapter.

One of the most prominent areas of concern is the tension that exists between the need to conduct HIV testing programs and the Anglo-Saxon legal tradition, which confers on individuals a strong right to privacy, particularly in matters such as sexual behavior.[5] Critics of mandatory testing are especially concerned with the fact that confidentiality of test results cannot always be guaranteed. Such misgivings are certainly realistic. Test results are subject to court subpoena, for example. They can also be misused by unscrupulous persons who might employ them for purposes of blackmail. There is always a risk that supposedly confidential test records might be lost, as actually happened in Washington, D.C., where a log containing the names of 500 people who had been tested for exposure to the AIDS virus was either lost or stolen.[6] Finally, there is the incipient worry that if extensive lists of HIV-infected people are compiled by public health authorities, they may ultimately be used by other government agencies in furtherance of various unpleasant political scenarios. That this fear is not an utter exaggeration can be seen in an order by the U.S. Department of Defense requiring civilian blood banks to disclose the names of active duty personnel who were found to be HIV-positive in blood donor screening.[7]

These concerns are important. If someone's seropositive status becomes known, he or she may be denied insurance, fired, evicted from rented housing, threatened with loss of child custody in divorce proceedings, or even physically assaulted. However, despite such possible negative consequences, mandatory testing programs are completely legal and constitutional. As the Yale AIDS Law Project puts it,

> ... screening by public health officials has traditionally been accepted by the courts as a valid public health measure. While the Supreme Court has recognized the importance of maintaining the confidentiality of medical data, it has also made very clear its faith in the confidentiality protections provided in typical health laws.[8]

Futhermore, while in the past seropositivity was often equated with homosexuality or illicit drug use, such "automatic" stigmatization will be greatly reduced now that HIV infection is clearly spreading beyond the original high-risk groups into the general population.

Given this analysis, it is fair to say that the confidentiality issue is largely a matter of perspective. In fact, existing public health laws on the confidentiality of medical test data fully meet all constitutional requirements for protecting privacy. This may be in part why civil rights proponents have been remarkably silent about the confidentiality of HIV test data gathered routinely in blood donor screening programs. (Blood banks not only maintain computerized lists of people who have tested positive, they exchange this information with other blood banks.) If these programs have managed to do a reasonable job of maintaining confidentiality, why isn't it likely that public health programs will be able to do at least as good a job?

Another aspect of the civil rights issue relates to people who are tested and have a false positive result (that is, one that identifies them as infected with the AIDS virus when they are not). It can be argued that persons who subject themselves to voluntary testing do so understanding in advance that such testing will yield a small but significant number of false positive results; in a sense, then, if they agree to have such a test performed, they also agree to accept this risk. Though they will experience the negative effects of such a mistake, it would not appear that their civil rights have been violated. However, for those who are not tested voluntarily, the stigma, psychological trauma, and other serious ramifications (e.g., a woman in this category deciding not to become pregnant or deciding to have an abortion if she is pregnant) are both immeasurable and a direct civil rights infringement, apparently as a by-product of compliance with a legislative act. In a country where concern over the privacy of sexual matters is so great "that an untrue allegation that someone has a venereal disease can lead to recovery of monetary damages for slander per se or defamation," and where the California Supreme Court allowed a lawsuit against a hospital that mistakenly diagnosed a woman as having syphilis,[9] the enormity of the impact that thousands of such false positive results will have is definitely not something to be taken lightly. (Later in this chapter we will suggest a partial remedy for this situation.)

Nevertheless, it is also evident that the AIDS epidemic may claim millions of lives. Especially given the rather dim prospects at present for a vaccine or a cure,[10] it seems of paramount importance to rapidly implement a rational, systematic effort to limit the spread of the virus. We believe that the type of testing, reporting, and contact tracing programs we will recommend actually do more on balance to *preserve* civil rights than to weaken them. With adequate attention to the details of providing the maximum degree of confidentiality possible—both legislatively and in the actual administration of public health departments and testing laboratories—and with further refinements in testing techniques that will reduce the number of false positive tests (which is currently thought to be only 1 in 10,000),[11] we can keep disruptions of civil liberties to a minimum while significantly increasing our vigilance against a lethal disease that could prove to be the worst natural calamity of this century.

While we are on the subject of civil rights, we should point to two specific instances where we believe the civil rights banner has no business at all being waved. It is both puzzling and distressing to see that in a number of locations, including New York City, homosexual bathhouses are still in operation.[12] The basic contention of those who advocate keeping the gay bathhouses open is that they serve as education centers, reaching an audience that otherwise wouldn't receive adequate public health warnings about high-risk sexual behavior. This notion—bathhouse as institute of higher learning—is totally nonsensical since the primary purpose of the gay baths has long been to provide a meeting place for anonymous sexual encounters.[13] In fact, despite periodic claims to the contrary in the press, high-risk sex (anal intercourse and oral sex without use of condoms) is the primary activity occurring in the private cubicles of these bathhouses, and the major reason they remain open is economic, not philosophical.[14]

Far more people are placed at risk by the ready availability of prostitutes in most metropolitan areas. Since very high numbers of prostitutes are now carriers of the AIDS virus,[15] it is difficult to understand why anyone would be willing to utilize their services, but it is clear that they are still in great demand. Under the circumstances, it seems important to acknowledge that—right now, at least—prostitution is not, in fact, a "victimless crime," and to strongly urge governmental crackdowns on prostitution. While we might sympathize with the economic plight of prostitutes who can no longer earn a living in their chosen occupation, this sympathy shouldn't lead us to act differently than we do when we take away the flight license of an airline pilot who has a medical condition that might jeopardize the lives of his passengers. There is certainly ample public health documentation, both in the U.S. and abroad, that regulation of prostitution is an important step in slowing the spread of sexually transmitted diseases.[16]

MANDATORY TESTING FOR HIV: SPECIAL POPULATIONS

Mandatory HIV antibody testing programs have already been implemented in several population groups: blood donors, U.S. military personnel and recruits, prisoners in federal penitentiaries, and immigrants to the United States.[17] Such programs have a threefold purpose. They allow collection of epidemiologic data that help describe current patterns of HIV infection and are necessary for projections about future trends. They serve a preventive function by identifying infected people and counseling them about how to avoid transmitting the infection to others. (Screening blood donors, of course, provides a different type of prevention by reducing the number of units of infected blood that enter the nation's blood supply.) In addition, testing programs can afford an opportunity to trace the sex and drug contacts of infected persons, leading to the discovery of further cases of infection and the chance to counsel uninfected people whose behavior puts them at risk for infection.

We believe that mandatory HIV testing programs should be expanded to include several additional population groups now, before the prevalence of HIV infection rises much higher. These groups should be: (1) pregnant women; (2) anyone between the ages of 15 and 60 admitted to a hospital; (3) convicted prostitutes; and (4) all marriage license applicants.

The case for testing pregnant women is especially compelling. Since there is mounting evidence that infection with the AIDS virus has escalated among heterosexuals,[18] since it is clear that in women the infection is most common during their reproductive years,[19] and since 50% or more of babies born to infected women will be infected with the AIDS virus,[20] not to perform such testing on a mandatory basis is a matter of medical irresponsibility. The urgency of the situation is shown by data from several recent surveys of pregnant women. In Massachusetts, where the State Department of Health screened blood specimens obtained from 14,699 newborn babies between December 1986 and April 1987, it was found that the prevalence of HIV infection among pregnant women was 230 per 100,000[21]—a level approximately four times as high as found in female military recruits. In a prenatal clinic in Jacksonville, Florida—a city not known for high rates of AIDS—a voluntary screening program showed a prevalence rate of 670 per 100,000 for HIV antibody seropositivity among pregnant women.[22] And at an inner city municipal hospital in New York, a recent study found that 12 of 602 pregnant women were seropositive,[23] which is a prevalence rate of about 2,000 per 100,000. This study also cited unpublished data from Bellevue Hospital in New York showing a seroprevalence rate of

3.7%—3,700 per 100,000—among women who had just given birth.

While it is certainly true that many pregnant women who are seropositive may decide to continue their pregnancies rather than abort them,[24] we believe every woman so affected should be given this choice—and she cannot be given the choice without prenatal screening for HIV infection. At the same time, we strongly oppose any legislative attempts either to mandate abortions for pregnant HIV-infected women or to prohibit pregnancy in infected women, if only because it is possible that 50% of the children born to these women will *not* be infected.

A mandatory hospital admissions screening program for anyone between the ages of 15 and 60* would be valuable for a number of reasons. Several studies done on groups of hospital admissions or emergency room patients have already uncovered an unexpectedly high prevalence of HIV infection.[25] A compulsory testing program would provide much-needed epidemiological information for tracking broad population trends of HIV infection, which would have important implications for public health planning. Such screening would also provide important medical information pertinent to the care of each patient. For instance, patients who are infected with HIV may have adverse responses to certain vaccines or may require special regimens of treatment for other-

*This age range currently includes the great majority of people at risk; however, once the cost effectiveness of such a program is demonstrated, and as more epidemiologic information becomes available, it may prove most effective to broaden the age range or even screen all hospital admissions.

157

wise routinely treated conditions.[26] Furthermore, it is important to avoid exposing HIV-infected patients, whose immunity is likely to be depressed, to other patients with contagious illnesses. Thus, there are sound medical reasons for identifying patients with HIV infection that have to do with the treatment and well-being of the patient.

In addition, since HIV can be transmitted via skin contact with biological fluids from infected persons,[27] it is imperative that health care workers and ancillary hospital personnel (e.g., maids; kitchen aides who pick up used dishes, trays, and eating utensils; laundry workers who might handle soiled linens) be alerted to the risks of exposure (which are, of course, particularly heightened for members of surgical teams or for those administering injections or performing invasive procedures of any sort). It is certainly apparent to anyone familiar with practices in most hospitals at present that the CDC's guidelines for precautions to be used in coming in contact with patients' biological fluids are not being followed by most personnel with any degree of consistency. Furthermore, it is not difficult to envision a scene in which a patient who is sharing a semiprivate room with someone whose HIV-positive status is undetected might inadvertently use the infected person's toothbrush or razor, or come in contact with infected blood or saliva by a small act of kindness—helping to change a bandage or wiping the person's face with a napkin or washcloth.

With regard to mandatory HIV screening for hospital admissions, it is relevant to note that from the late 1930s on, admissions orders at virtually every hospital in the United States routinely instructed that all patients be tested for syphilis, regardless of age. (This requirement was at one time so stringent that if a patient was discharged from the hospital a day after admission and was readmitted just a few days later, it was necessary to repeat the test.) While this program was begun voluntarily by hospitals and physicians as a means of controlling what was then called venereal disease, unlimited free blood testing services were provided by state health department laboratories.[28] The program (in conjunction with other mandatory testing programs) was so successful in reducing the prevalence of syphilis that in 1955 the American Hospital Association dropped routine serologic screening as a requirement for hospital accreditation, although the vast majority of hospitals and physicians continued to screen virtually all hospital admissions and new patients as they had before.[29] The tests used for such screening had a substantial number of false positives (far higher than the number found with HIV antibody testing), but this mandatory testing program did not seem to pose much of a threat to anyone's civil rights and did not result in major breaches of patient confidentiality either.

The rationale behind a mandatory testing program for convicted prostitutes should be obvious. There are already high rates of HIV infection in prostitutes in many major American cities.[30] It is difficult to imagine a group in which the risk of sexual transmission is any greater, since most prostitutes have astonishing numbers of customers in the course of a year. In addition, as we mentioned in an earlier chapter, a sizable number of prostitutes are drug addicts, which means that they are likely to be transmitting the virus by the sharing of con-

159

taminated needles and syringes. Not to conduct mandatory testing in this group would be absurd: after all, if a prostitute has been arrested, tried, and convicted (or pleads guilty to the charges), confidentiality regarding the fact that he or she has engaged in prostitution has already evaporated.

MANDATORY PREMARITAL TESTING
FOR HIV

One of the most hotly debated of possible public policies to contain the AIDS epidemic is a compulsory national premarital screening program. Among the various objections to such a policy, the most compelling is a practical one: that it would be an ineffective and inefficient use of resources. Precisely this conclusion was reached in late 1987 by a group from the Division of Health Policy Research at Harvard University.[31] Because of the importance of the issue, we will summarize the details of the Harvard Study Group's analysis and then offer a critique of their calculations and conclusions (for the statistics and computations behind our critique, see Appendix C).

The Harvard team began with data taken from U.S. government vital statistics for 1982, during which year 1,912,684 marriages occurred in this country (Table 9.1). They assumed—on the basis of prevalence figures from various blood donor screening programs—"that men between the ages of 18 and 45 would have a prevalence of HIV infection of 70 per 100,000 and that all others have a rate of seven per 100,000."[32] Next they assumed that the

TABLE 9.1
Number of Persons Married in 1982

AGE RANGE (YRS.)	WOMEN	MEN
14–17	84,943	12,818
18–19	255,254	119,652
20–24	685,773	632,089
25–29	395,910	477,761
30–34	201,921	258,802
35–44	171,884	228,931
45–64	98,706	148,767
≥ 65	18,293	33,864
Total	1,912,684	1,912,684

Source: U.S. Department of Health and Human Services, *Vital Statistics of the United States: 1982,* vol. 3, *Marriage and Divorce.* These data served as the basis for the analysis conducted by the Harvard Study Group: "Compulsory Premarital Screening for the Human Immunodeficiency Virus: Technical and Public Health Considerations," *Journal of the American Medical Association* 258: 1757–62, 1987.

sensitivity and specificity of the ELISA test for HIV antibodies would be 98.3% and 99.8% respectively, while the Western blot test used to check all specimens that were repeatedly positive with the ELISA test would have a sensitivity of 92% and a specificity of 95%. They also assumed that 60% of the couples getting married would have engaged in premarital sexual intercourse before screening, and that where one partner was infected with the AIDS virus, the rate of sexual transmission to the other, previously uninfected partner would be 10%.

Working from these assumptions, the Harvard group estimated that previously undetected seropositive status would be discovered in about 1,200 people as a result of

3.8 million ELISA tests done for premarital screening, with an additional 10,000 Western blot tests required for confirmatory purposes. They noted that such testing would cost approximately $23 million and would need to be supplemented with counseling services at an additional cost of more than $100 million. Comparing costs with results, they concluded that the program would prove both inefficient and ineffective. We agree with the general framework of their analysis but not with the conclusion, since we can show that several of the assumptions on which it is based are seriously flawed.

A key issue is the Harvard Study Group's assumption that the prevalence of HIV infection in the population getting married is identical to the prevalence in a population of blood donors. This assumption is incorrect for several reasons. First, 46.8% of those getting married in 1982 were in the 14-to-24-year-old age bracket. This is considerably different from the age distribution in the blood donor population. Second, it is well known that persons who have had hepatitis B or are carriers of the hepatitis B virus are not permitted to give blood. Because homosexual men and IV drug abusers—the two groups in which the prevalence of hepatitis B virus infection is highest[33]—are apt to be aware of this policy, many of them do not volunteer to be blood donors, which artificially reduces the prevalence rate for HIV infection found in blood donor screening programs as compared to the population at large. (This effect may have become more pronounced in recent years as homosexual or bisexual males have learned that blood banks will actively exclude anyone who admits to a history of same-sex behavior.) Third, pregnant women are not likely to be blood donors, although clearly a significant number of pregnant women are infected with the AIDS virus[34] and clearly many pregnant women are also in the group applying for marriage licenses, as the Harvard Study Group acknowledges.[35]

At the least, it would appear that the Harvard team should have used prevalence figures from the U.S. military screening program to apply to the younger persons who comprised almost half of the hypothetical population in their model: these figures—which are based on tests of more than 3 million people, both recruits and active duty personnel—are 160 per 100,000 for males and 60 per 100,000 for females.[36] However, even these statistics probably understate the actual prevalence in the population at large, and in the population applying for marriage licenses, because homosexual and bisexual men are actively discouraged from joining the military yet a significant number of them actually get married. While this assertion might seem surprising at first glance, the research evidence to back it up is formidable. For instance, Bell and Weinberg reported that 20% of the white homosexual men (N = 575) and 13% of the black homosexual men in their sample (N = 111) had been married.[37] Other studies have reported comparable findings.[38] Similarly, it is unlikely that many drug addicts, either male or female, sign on with the military, yet there are clearly drug addicts among people applying for marriage licenses.

In addition, it appears that the Harvard Study Group seriously underestimated the prevalence of HIV infection among women of reproductive age. Not only is the prevalence figure they used for their calculations (7 per

100,000) far below that found in female military recruits (60 per 100,000), it is also substantially lower than the prevalence rate determined in other studies. A case in point is the previously cited study by investigators at the Massachusetts Department of Health, who estimated that the HIV antibody prevalence rate among women of childbearing age in Massachusetts is 230 per 100,000.[39] In New York City an estimated 3% (3,000 per 100,000) of women of reproductive age are HIV carriers.[40]

We believe that the Harvard Study Group's prevalence figures for HIV infection should be modified to correct for these realities as follows: for the population of women age 34 and under, we would apply a figure of 60 per 100,000; for 95% of the population of men age 44 and under, we would apply the baseline prevalence rate of 160 per 100,000 found by the military screening program; and we would adjust for the 5% of men getting married who might reasonably be expected to be homosexual, bisexual, or IV drug users, applying to this group a very conservative prevalence figure of 10,000 per 100,000.* If we make only these adjustments, the conclusions of the Harvard Study Group are altered considerably, as we show in Table 9.2. The result is that

*Most studies have found that among homosexual and bisexual men, the prevalence of HIV infection ranges from 50% to 75% depending on where the sample population is obtained. Among IV drug abusers, "published estimates of infection range from a low of 9% . . . to 64%," according to the authoritative report of the Institute of Medicine and National Academy of Sciences. Thus, our assumption of a 10% prevalence rate of HIV infection in the population of gay, bisexual, and IV drug-using men who marry each year is indeed a very conservative one; if the actual prevalence is substantially more than this, it would raise our calculated results considerably.

TABLE 9.2
**Mandatory Premarital Screening: Number of Persons Estimated
to Be Infected, by Age and Gender, Harvard Study Group
Prevalence Assumptions Versus Modified Prevalence
Assumptions**[a]

AGE RANGE (YRS.)	INFECTED FEMALES		INFECTED MALES	
	Estimated # from Baseline Prevalence			
14–17	51	*6*	84	*1*
18–19	153	*18*	780	*84*
20–24	411	*48*	4,122	*442*
25–34	238	*28*	3,114	*334*
30–34	121	*14*	1,687	*181*
35–44	12	*12*	1,493	*160*
45–64	7	*7*	10	*10*
≥ 65	1	*1*	2	*2*
Subtotal	994	*134*	11,292	*1,214*
	Estimated # Infected by Partner[b]			
	678	—	60	—
Total	1,672	—	11,352	—

[a]Assumptions as stated in text; Harvard Study Group estimates in italics.

[b]The Harvard Study Group did not break these computations down in their
report but estimated that there would have been approximately 70 cases of
HIV transmission from an infected partner.

approximately 13,000 cases of HIV infection would be
detected in the first year of a national premarital screening program, rather than the 1,200 claimed in the Harvard Study Group's report.

More important, since HIV infection is known to be a
lifetime condition, the prevalence in the general population mounts as new infections occur (that is, at least until
the annual death rate of persons infected with HIV ex-

ceeds the number of new cases each year). Thus, in subsequent years the yield of such a mandatory premarital
testing program, measured in numbers of infected individuals identified, would be expected to increase substantially.

This is not just an academic exercise. A mandatory
premarital testing program for infection with the AIDS
virus is important for a number of reasons. First, identifying cases of HIV infection premaritally gives prospective spouses the opportunity to decline to marry. In
effect, it is a full-disclosure policy that permits both partners to give informed consent rather than entering the
marriage contract without a key piece of information that
may have serious economic, health, reproductive, and
psychological ramifications. Second, if a woman is infected with the AIDS virus, the couple should know that
if they plan to have children, there is a high potential of
having an infected baby. While this will not prevent all
pregnancy-transmitted infections, it is logical to assume
that it will reduce the incidence of this human tragedy.
(Based on our calculations, close to 6,000 infected births
might be prevented by just one year of mandatory
premarital screening.) Third, the epidemiological data
gathered in such a mandatory screening program would
provide the scientific and public health community, as
well as legislators, with much more accurate information
on trends in the AIDS epidemic among people who are
apparently healthy. Such information is far more valuable from an epidemiologic point of view than data about
hospitalized patients, so even if a mandatory hospital
admissions testing program were to be established, it
would not diminish the importance of premarital testing

as a public health tool. Without such broad-based national data—which are unlikely to be obtained in any voluntary testing program—effective planning about the epidemic is virtually impossible, as we have already seen, much to the regret of many scientists and government officials.

Precisely this point was made by various expert witnesses testifying before Congress in August 1987 during hearings on several bills to provide federal funding for widespread testing programs. For instance, Dr. Robert R. Redfield, who is one of the U.S. Army's top AIDS researchers, declared that it is "critical" to shift our current focus from AIDS as a full-blown disease to patterns of transmission of the AIDS virus. Dr. Redfield noted that if the emphasis remains on actual cases of AIDS, "we are doomed to failure because the magnitude of our response is a decade out of sync." He strongly urged the priority of testing programs that would inform public health authorities about the epidemiology of viral transmission today and help prevent further spread of the virus by asymptomatic carriers who don't realize they're infected.[41]

Apart from claims of inefficiency, there are three other frequent objections to the idea of mandatory premarital testing for the AIDS virus. The first is that a mandatory testing program will frighten off a disproportionate number of high-risk persons, thereby keeping them from being tested and discovering that they are infected. The second objection is that mandatory as opposed to voluntary testing is an infringement of civil rights, particularly the right to privacy. The third is that as a result of inherent inaccuracies in current antibody testing methods, a

167

number of people will have false positive results and will be mistakenly told that they are carriers of the AIDS virus. Let us consider each of these objections a bit further.

It is probably true that some people will avoid marriage because they do not want to be tested for the AIDS virus, but it is hard to predict exactly how many. We believe that it is highly improbable that even 1% of the pool of potential marriage applicants would decide not to marry just to avoid being tested. From a public health viewpoint, a program that managed to test 99% of the population it was intended to screen would be a resounding success. If some individuals already know from prior anonymous testing that they are infected and decide that they won't attempt to marry, this will not interfere with the program and in some ways may actually help to achieve the same end result. In fact, if a mandatory premarital testing program is implemented, as we are urging, anyone who senses that a partner's reluctance to marry might be related to fear of being tested would probably be justified in asking the partner to be tested voluntarily (as outlined in Chapter 7) before agreeing to have intimate sexual contact.

The civil rights issue is not, in our minds, a major stumbling block when it comes to compulsory premarital testing, partly for reasons discussed previously. In addition, of course, most states have a long history of requiring premarital blood tests for syphilis.[42] Although some states have dropped these requirements for economic reasons, there has been little objection in the past to premarital testing as an issue of civil rights. It seems to us that the risks associated with HIV infection are so great that it is a violation of civil rights *not* to utilize the available screening technology, which is reasonably sophisticated and sensitive although not perfect, just as syphilis testing methods are not foolproof. That is, a value must be assigned to the health of the prospective marriage partner (and of unborn children). At the very least, everyone has a right to be informed whether his or her prospective partner has a sexually transmissable, untreatable, generally lethal infection.

The objection to mandatory premarital testing because of a small number of false positive test results seems to us misguided. It is certainly true that such false positives will occur. The Harvard Study Group estimated that there would be 382 false positives (out of 3.8 million tests) in the first year of mandatory premarital screening,[43] and it is clear that the lives of these people and their prospective spouses would be affected in serious ways. Some women (or couples) might decide not to have children and might even undergo voluntary sterilization in order to be sure of preventing conception. Equally tragically, some couples might decide not to marry on the basis of the erroneous information. It is even possible that a person incorrectly labeled HIV-positive might commit suicide as a result of the severe psychological strain attendant upon such a diagnosis. However, the number of false positive results must be looked at in a broader context: that of the number of infected persons accurately identified by such a testing program and of the several million people who will be correctly informed that they are free of HIV infection. For many in the latter group, a negative test result may provide strong motivation for risk-free sexual behav-

169

ior—so that testing becomes, in effect, a catalyst for maintenance of sound public health practices. Even more important, those who discover that they are infected with the AIDS virus can be offered individualized counseling by specially trained public health personnel to guide them in directions that should help to contain the spread of the infection. This, after all, is what such testing is about.

One should never disregard the undeserved anguish and suffering of those few people who are inadvertently hurt by public policy decisions aimed at the so-called greater good. There is also, of course, the danger that the "greater good" may be so nebulous or even noxious a concept that it has no applicability in a given set of circumstances. Here, in the face of an epidemic that is clearly raging uncontrolled at present and that is expected to take millions of lives worldwide unless its spread is quickly checked, we must define the greater good specifically in public health terms, and we must be prepared to deal with its casualties. Therefore, federal and state agencies should set up a special fund to provide reparations to persons who are later found to have been erroneously diagnosed as HIV antibody-positive. Every possible scientific effort should be put into improving the accuracy of current test methods and developing new testing technologies that will materially reduce the number of false positive results. But to allow tens of thousands of cases of HIV infection (if not more) to go undetected because of delays in implementing a national testing program is to abdicate our responsibility to the public welfare, just as delaying the introduction of polio vaccine in the 1950s would have been unconscionable even in the face of problems and uncertainties (including a small number of polio cases actually transmitted by the vaccines).

Two last points should be made about mandatory premarital screening and false positive results. First, it is interesting to see that no one is insisting that the blood supply shouldn't be screened because of the problem of too many false positives. Yet the percentage of false positive errors in screening blood donors is precisely the same as it would be in a mandatory premarital HIV testing program (because exactly the same laboratory tests with exactly the same sources of error would be used). Second, as the prevalence of HIV infection increases in the general population, as it inevitably must do over time until a vaccine is found, the relative number of false positive tests will decrease.[44] This general principle of screening programs is of particular importance because the need for mandatory premarital testing will be even more acute if the prevalence of infection in the general population becomes considerably higher than it is today. We are afraid that this is exactly what is going to happen. Playing ostrich in the face of this reality is not going to save lives or diminish the anguish in our world—in fact, it will have precisely the opposite effect.

MANDATORY REPORTING OF HIV INFECTION

We believe that it is essential to go beyond the point of only requiring that AIDS cases (as opposed to cases of

171

infection with the AIDS virus) be reported to public health authorities, as though AIDS (the disease) were more important from a preventive viewpoint than infection with the AIDS virus. Unless state legislatures—or Congress—tackle this issue quickly, we will reach a point where HIV infection is so widespread that containment measures are virtually guaranteed to be ineffective. The result, eventually, will be millions of unnecessary deaths.

If *all* states adopt mandatory reporting laws in conjunction with mandatory premarital screening and mandatory testing of all hospitalized patients, it is unlikely that many people will be driven away by fear of having a positive test reported to the authorities. Indeed, most people will realize that the broader the testing programs, the less the chance of any single group of infected persons being targeted for discriminatory action. This will be particularly true, in our judgment, as the prevalence of AIDS infection escalates over the next five to ten years.

CONTACT TRACING AND NOTIFICATION

It seems anomalous, but the single most useful means of identifying people infected with the AIDS virus has been almost completely ignored in the nation's current response to the AIDS crisis. Contact tracing, which involves identifying, notifying, testing, and counseling people who have had sexual contact (or have shared needles) with someone known to be infected, has been assiduously avoided in most states, although Colorado and Louisiana are current exceptions to this generalization.

Tracking the sex partners of people with reportable sexually transmitted diseases has been employed for many decades as a public health strategy.[45] Because it provides a targeted approach to case detection, focusing on people with a high probability of exposure, it is highly efficient in identifying individuals with previously undetected infection. In addition to its value as a numerical exercise, contact tracing is important as a means of reducing the rate of spread of infection: by identifying people who don't suspect that they might be infected, testing them, and providing them with appropriate counseling, this technique is likely to have considerable preventive impact.

Various objections have been raised to the idea of using routine contact tracing at this stage in the AIDS epidemic. For instance, some opponents of this strategy have pointed out that contact tracing programs may encourage anonymous sexual encounters among people who are afraid that if they can be identified by their partners, their names may be given to public health authorities.[46] Others insist that contact tracing programs require absolute confidentiality but that such confidentiality cannot be guaranteed since legislative changes or court subpoenas can ordinarily pierce the protective shield. Furthermore, if contact tracing is initiated, will it stop with notification, testing, and counseling, or will it (and should it) eventually lead to follow-up investigations to determine, for example, whether infected persons are continuing to participate in unsafe sex—with possible criminal charges to be brought against them if

173

they are? In addition to these concerns, others point out that the expense of a comprehensive contact tracing program is likely to be prohibitive, especially in the states where HIV prevalence rates are highest.

Certainly these are important concerns. No contact tracing program will be able to offer absolute guarantees that there will not be some problems. However, we believe that these problems would be significantly outweighed by the benefits deriving from notification of unsuspecting infected individuals and the concomitant slowing of the spread of infection. In fact, the very worry about the possibility of being traced that may drive some people to anonymous sex will probably act as a deterrent for many others, causing them to think twice before putting themselves in sexual situations that might expose them to the AIDS virus.

There is another aspect to this issue that has been more or less brushed under the rug until recently. If a physician or other health care worker knows that a male patient is infected with the AIDS virus and hasn't told his wife (or vice versa), isn't there a duty to warn her even if the husband objects? If the couple is having unprotected sex or considering a pregnancy, shouldn't the physician's duty to notify the wife be even more compelling? There have been some court decisions suggesting that the physician does indeed have a duty to warn in these sorts of circumstances, but without contact tracing and notification laws, many physicians may feel unable to do so on the grounds that such an act would be a violation of patient confidentiality.[47]

We have already shown that the efforts mounted to

date have done far less to slow the spread of the AIDS epidemic than the public has realized. Educational campaigns by themselves, even on a much more comprehensive scale than has been tried up until now, will not stop risky sexual behavior. Even mandatory testing programs, which will provide a major impetus toward change, will not insure the highest degree of public health safety that we can attain. In light of the price that must be paid in human suffering and lives if this epidemic is not contained within the next two years, the need for a contact tracing program seems compelling.

IS QUARANTINE NECESSARY?

The fears provoked by the AIDS epidemic have inevitably raised the specter of quarantine as a social policy issue. In Cuba such a policy has already been instituted— 108 people infected with the AIDS virus have been sequestered on a farm outside Havana—and in a few isolated cases, primarily involving infected prostitutes, courts in the United States have issued quarantine orders.[48]

At one level the issue seems very simple. There can be no justification for imposing quarantine on infected persons who do not continue to expose others to their infection. Since we are not dealing with a virus that is transmitted by the airborne route or by mere proximity to an infected person, the risk of transmission is primarily (but not solely) restricted to sex partners and those who share needles and syringes with an infected person. On the other hand, it is clear to everyone working in the field that there are thousands of HIV-infected people who know their status and continue to have multiple sexual contacts, often without revealing that they are carriers of the virus (which might, understandably, cause their partners to rethink the wisdom of the liaison). There are also tens of thousands of infected drug users who continue to share needles and syringes with others (although it is less certain that an addict will decline the invitation to share, even knowing the risk of infection). What should be done to deal with these cases? What should be done to protect the public against prostitutes, male and female, who are infected with the AIDS virus and continue to ply their trade? What should be done about someone who knows that he or she is infected but still tries to donate blood? What about someone with AIDS who bites a police officer?

Quarantine is not a reasonable answer to these difficult questions. It seems more appropriate at this juncture to deal with such cases as matters of criminal law. Clearly, just as the constitutional guarantees of freedom of speech do not (and should not) extend to someone falsely yelling "Fire" in a crowded theater, constitutional guarantees of privacy should not permit anyone to knowingly endanger the life of another person by willful conduct that might be considered a form of attempted murder. Since very few legal precedents exist in this area, the situation regarding such behavior is much murkier than it should be.

Though a number of states have old laws on their books that prohibit knowingly transmitting a venereal disease, in most cases these laws have not been updated to classify AIDS as a venereal disease. New legislation is required to modernize this entire area of law and give courts the power to imprison persons whose persistent irresponsible behavior exposes others to infection with the AIDS virus. Such laws would no more infringe individual civil rights than laws that prohibit stealing infringe the civil rights of bank robbers. When the act in question is as clearly harmful as transmission of the AIDS virus, there should be no equivocating.[49]

A CONCLUDING NOTE

Governments across the world will have to struggle with many difficult questions in confronting the realities of the AIDS epidemic. May their attempt to find answers be informed by a wise balance between compassion, rationality, and adequate protection of the public health.

We have already witnessed a distressingly slow response to the AIDS epidemic in America and in the world at large. It is quite clear today, as it has been from the inception of this epidemic, that not enough money has been earmarked for research. It is also quite clear that not enough attention has been paid to the fact that the AIDS virus infects people regardless of their sexual orientation, their morals, or their age. While we fervently hope that mindless panic over the AIDS epidemic will not dictate government policies, we are also convinced that if implementation of effective prevention strategies is delayed by a mistaken belief that this epi-

APPENDIX A
CLINICAL FEATURES OF AIDS

AIDS is the end stage of HIV infection. Although it occurs primarily among men aged 20 to 40, it has been documented in all age groups and in a growing number of women. With more than 45,000 cases reported in the U.S. by late 1987—and more than 100,000 cases worldwide—this disease is truly growing in epidemic proportions.

The precise definition of AIDS used for "official" purposes (that is, for national surveillance and reporting) was first established by the CDC in 1982 (CDC, Update on acquired immune deficiency syndrome [AIDS]—United States, *Morbidity and Mortality Weekly Report* 31: 507–14, 1982). According to this definition, AIDS could only be diagnosed in the presence of another disease—such as *Pneumocystis carinii* pneumonia, a previously rare type of lung infection, or Kaposi's sarcoma, an unusual form of cancer of the small blood vessels—that generally occurred only in the presence of disruption of the immune system. In addition, the CDC definition required that in such cases, the immune deficiency was not the result of medications, certain forms of cancer, or other known causes such as an inborn defect in the production of antibodies (substances produced by the immune system to fight off invasion by infecting organisms or other "foreign" intruders into the body). Following the discovery of HIV and the development of tests to detect HIV antibody, the CDC's definition was expanded in 1985 to include certain other so-called opportunistic infections and cancers of the lymph tissue in people who were found to be infected with HIV or to test positive for HIV antibodies (*MMWR* 34: 373–75, 1985). This definition was revised and expanded again in late 1987 (*MMWR* 36, Supplement 1S, 1987).

Setting aside the precise requirements of the CDC's diagnostic criteria, there are several different categories of illness that are apt to make up the clinical constellation we know as AIDS. No precise pattern of symptoms fits all cases. The most typical early findings are progressive unexplained weight loss, persistent fever, and swollen lymph nodes. These nonspecific symptoms may occur in a person who otherwise feels completely healthy or may be accompanied by a sense of feeling rundown or sick. The earliest symptoms may completely disappear in a few cases, may remain bothersome but unchanged for many months, or may quickly be followed by one or more unusual forms of infection.

The most important of these is a group of infections known as opportunistic infections. The term "opportunistic" indicates that these particular infections rarely occur in the absence of some factor that suppresses the immune system. In other words, these infections typically require a special opportunity—a relatively immobilized immune response—to successfully invade the body and create illness. Under ordinary circumstances, when the immune system is functioning normally, the body's natural defenses are almost always able to repel an assault by these microbial pathogens.

Here is a list summarizing the main opportunistic infections that are found among people with AIDS:

- *Pneumocystis carinii* pneumonia—an especially virulent form of previously rare pneumonia that is the

most common AIDS-related infection; it usually
presents with fever, cough, shortness of breath (especially with exertion), and tightness in the chest;

* chronic cryptosporidiosis and isosporiasis—two
related parasites that produce a self-limited diarrhea in normal hosts but lead to profuse diarrhea,
malnutrition, and severe weight loss in AIDS patients;

* toxoplasmosis—an infection caused by *Toxoplasma
gondii,* which produces a wide variety of neurologic
abnormalities in AIDS patients, including seizures
and encephalopathy, as well as infections of the
heart and lungs;

* extraintestinal strongyloidiasis—a parasitic infection that can produce damage to the lungs as well
as meningitis;

* candidiasis—a fungus infection that in its mildest
forms causes thrush or vaginitis but in its disseminated form can cause painful infections of the
esophagus;

* cryptococcosis—a fungus infection that commonly
causes meningitis in AIDS patients and can also infect the lungs;

* disseminated histoplasmosis—a usually mild fungus
infection that in AIDS patients can cause pneumonia, hepatitis, adrenal insufficiency, infections of the
heart valves, and meningitis;

* mycobacterial infections—unusual forms of myco-
bacteria, such as *M. avian* and *M. kansasii,* often
cause fever, wasting, and fatigue;

* disseminated cytomegalovirus infection—an infection caused by a common virus that is usually harm-

less in people with normal immune systems but in AIDS patients spreads widely throughout the body, causing painful esophagitis, colitis, dementia (because of encephalopathy), pneumonia, and infections of the retina that, untreated, lead to blindness;

- chronic mucocutaneous or disseminated herpes simplex virus infection—these not only may involve the skin, the mouth, and the eyes but may also cause encephalitis, myelitis, and pneumonia;
- progressive multifocal leukoencephalopathy—a rare, uniformly fatal neurologic condition that usually occurs in immunosuppressed patients; it causes symptoms such as hemiplegia, aphasia (inability to speak), and organic mental changes and typically follows a rapidly downhill course.

In addition, many people with HIV infection develop other infections that are not part of the CDC's diagnostic criteria, including:

oral hairy leukoplakia
multidermatomal herpes zoster (shingles)
recurrent *Salmonella* bacteremia
nocardiasis
tuberculosis
oral candidiasis (thrush)

In addition to opportunistic infections, opportunistic malignancies—forms of cancer that are relatively rare except in persons with suppressed immunity—occur with some frequency among people with AIDS. Kaposi's sarcoma, which typically appears as reddish-purple, raised, coin-sized bumps on the skin, is the most frequently found cancer of this type.

For reasons that are unclear, Kaposi's sarcoma affects homosexual men who have AIDS more often than others who have AIDS: overall, it is found in about a quarter of U.S. AIDS cases and one-third of those in Europe. Other cancers that commonly appear in people with AIDS include a previously rare type called Burkitt's lymphoma and a form of lymphoma (a cancer of the lymphatic tissue) that involves the brain.

Because brain cells can be damaged by HIV infection, people with AIDS also have a high incidence of certain neurological disorders. These disorders are often debilitating, severe, and progressive. The most commonly encountered neurological problem is AIDS dementia (a combination of memory loss, impaired thinking, and mental confusion), which occurs in the majority of cases (Navia et al., *Annals of Neurology* 19: 517–24, 1986; D. H. Gabuzda and M. S. Hirsch, Neurologic manifestations of infection with human immunodeficiency virus, *Annals of Internal Medicine* 107: 383–91, 1987). The cognitive impairment is often accompanied by both behavioral symptoms such as depression, apathy, and social withdrawal, and physical problems such as difficulty with balance, leg weakness, and tremor. In more severe cases, incontinence, seizures, and outright psychosis occur.

Acute encephalitis, or inflammation of the brain, is commonly caused in people with AIDS by a protozoan organism called *Toxoplasma gondii;* early signs of this condition include seizures, headache, fever, and confusion, which may gradually progress to frank coma. Unless promptly treated, this infection is virtually always fatal. An unusual form of self-limited meningitis (inflammation of the covering of the brain) is also found in AIDS patients, occurring in about 5% of cases. Peripheral neuropathies that typically involve either painful sensations caused by even a gentle touch or spontaneous sensations of numbness or tingling also occur in 30% to 50% of AIDS patients.

As AIDS progresses, its victims become increasingly weak and debilitated. In part, this may be a result of the severe emaciation that occurs. This condition is so prominent that in Africa AIDS is often called "slim"—a grim reflection of the profound wasting that leaves people looking like the gaunt, harrowed concentration camp victims we remember from newsreels. Weakness and debility late in the course of AIDS probably also reflects the enormous physical toll of fighting off repeated infections in a virtual struggle for survival, as well as the neurological damage described above.

Based on current statistics, the average time of survival for people with AIDS is about two years after diagnosis. As a practical matter, this isn't a number that gives people with AIDS or their families much help: death sometimes comes quickly but at other times is a long-drawn-out process that may go on for three or four years or more. Recent projections suggest that 15% of AIDS patients will survive for 5 years (R. Rothenberg et al., Survival with the acquired immunodeficiency syndrome, *New England Journal of Medicine* 317: 1297–1302, 1987).

AIDS is an invariably fatal disease, at least as we know it today; while it is possible that we have seen the most severe cases of AIDS relatively early in the epidemic, with somewhat milder cases and lower mortality rates yet to come, the likelihood of such a shift seems pitifully small at present.

APPENDIX B
THE RESEARCH QUESTIONNAIRES

Recruitment of subjects for the study described in Chapter 4 was conducted simultaneously in New York, St. Louis, Atlanta, and Los Angeles beginning in February 1987. In each city, project personnel hired four to six persons to assist with the distribution of a brief letter explaining the existence of the project, accompanied by the short screening questionnaire reproduced below. These persons posted notices about the project in various locations (e.g., campus bulletin boards) and, more important, distributed screening questionnaires on-site at locations such as singles bars, singles dances, health clubs, and meetings of church and civic groups.

Nine hundred and twelve people responded to the posted notices with telephone calls asking about the project. Of this number, 634 (70%) completed the screening questionnaire. A total of 8,205 screening questionnaires was distributed on-site by paid project staff. Of these, 3,171 (39%) were completed and returned to us for processing. In each location, it took approximately four to five weeks to complete the screening process.

Appointments for the volunteers who met the study criteria were made by a project secretary in each location. Each volunteer then completed the research questionnaire, also reproduced below. Subjects were not paid for their participation.

Appendix B

The actual interviewing of subjects, which sought to clarify and expand on data given in answer to the research questionnaire, was carried out by Dr. Kolodny in New York and St. Louis and by project staff in Los Angeles and Atlanta. It took about seven to eight weeks of intensive work in each location to complete the actual data collection beyond the screening stage. All interviews and data collection were completed by early June 1987.

SCREENING QUESTIONNAIRE

ID # ⸺⸺⸺⸺⸺

1. Are you: Male   Female   (circle one)

2. What is your current age? ⸺⸺⸺⸺

3. What is your *current* marital status? (circle one only)

    A. Never married
    B. Engaged (currently)
    C. Married
    D. Divorced
    E. Remarried
    F. Widowed
    G. Separated
    H. Living with a man
    I. Living with a woman
    J. Other (explain) ⸺⸺⸺⸺⸺⸺⸺⸺⸺⸺⸺⸺

4. If you are currently married, what is the length of your marriage? ⸺⸺⸺⸺

5. If you are currently living with someone, how long has this relationship lasted? ⸺⸺⸺⸺

6. How many sex partners have you had in the preceding year? (circle one answer only)

A. None
B. One
C. Two or three
D. Four or five
E. Six to ten
F. Eleven or more

7. On average, how many sex partners have you had each year for the last five years? (circle one answer only)

   A. None
   B. One
   C. Two or three
   D. Four or five
   E. Six to ten
   F. Eleven or more

8. If you are married, engaged, or living with someone, do you think your partner has been completely faithful to you during the entire time of your relationship? (circle one response)

   A. Absolutely; I'm certain of this.
   B. Probably; I'm pretty sure, but not certain.
   C. Possibly; I think so, but I'm not too sure.
   D. Unlikely, but I don't know for a fact.
   E. No.

9. If you are married, engaged, or living with someone, have you been completely faithful to that person during the entire time of your relationship? (circle one response)

   A. Yes
   B. No

10. In the past ten years, have you had any sexual contact with a person of your same gender (a man with a man, or a woman with a woman)?

    A. Yes
    B. No

11. In the past ten years, have you received a blood transfusion?

    A. Yes
    B. No

12. Have you ever used a nonprescription drug by injection?

    A. Yes
    B. No

RESEARCH QUESTIONNAIRE

ID # _____ M/F _____ Date _____

PART I. DEMOGRAPHIC INFORMATION

1. What is your age? _____

2. What is your present occupation? _____

3. What is your *current* marital status? (circle one only)

    A. Never married
    B. Engaged (currently)
    C. Married
    D. Divorced
    E. Remarried
    F. Widowed
    G. Separated
    H. Living with a man
    I. Living with a woman
    J. Other (explain) _____

4. If you are currently married, what is the length of your marriage? _____

5. If you are currently living with someone, how long has this relationship lasted? _____

6. If you are currently divorced, how long has it been since your marriage ended? _____

7. What is your religious affiliation? (circle one answer only)

   A. Protestant
   B. Catholic
   C. Jewish
   D. None
   E. Other (please specify) _____

8. About how often do you attend church or synagogue?

   A. Daily or almost every day
   B. Three or four times a week
   C. Once or twice a week
   D. Two or three times a month
   E. Once a month
   F. Once every few months
   G. About once a year
   H. Less often than once a year
   I. Never

9. What is your race?

   A. White
   B. Black
   C. Hispanic
   D. Asian or Asian American
   E. Native American or Indian
   F. Other (please specify) _____

10. What is the highest level of education you have completed?

A. Doctoral level
B. Master's level
C. Graduate studies, but no degree
D. Four-year college
E. Two-year community college
F. Some college, but no degree
G. Technical, vocational, or trade school
H. High school
I. Some high school, but no degree
J. Other (please specify) ⎯⎯⎯⎯⎯⎯⎯⎯⎯⎯⎯⎯

11. Are you currently in school?

A. No
B. Yes, attending a graduate school
C. Yes, attending a four-year college
D. Yes, attending a two-year community college
E. Yes, attending a technical, vocational, or trade school
F. Other (please specify) ⎯⎯⎯⎯⎯⎯⎯⎯⎯⎯⎯⎯

12. Which of the following best describes your *own* total yearly income (not including a spouse's or partner's income)? Include all sources, such as wages, salaries, tips, interest and dividends, etc.

A. No income
B. Less than $2,500
C. $2,500 to $4,999
D. $5,000 to $7,499
E. $7,500 to $9,999
F. $10,000 to $14,999
G. $15,000 to $19,999
H. $20,000 to $24,999
I. $25,000 to $29,999
J. $30,000 to $49,999
K. $50,000 or more

PART II. MEDICAL INFORMATION

1. In the past ten years, have you been hospitalized for a medical illness?

   A. Yes
   B. No (If yes, please describe.) _____

2. In the past ten years, have you had any surgery?

   A. Yes
   B. No (If yes, please describe.) _____

3. In the past ten years, have you received a blood transfusion?

   A. Yes
   B. No

4. Have you ever been told that you had a venereal disease or sexually transmitted disease such as syphilis, gonorrhea, genital herpes, or chlamydia?

   A. Yes
   B. No (If yes, please describe.) _____

5. [Women only] Have you ever been pregnant?

   A. Yes
   B. No (If yes, how many times?) _____

6. How often do you use alcohol?

   A. Daily or almost daily
   B. Four or five times a week
   C. Two or three times a week
   D. Once a week
   E. One to three times a month
   F. A few times a year
   G. Less often than once a year
   H. Not at all

7. On occasions when you do use alcohol, how many drinks do you typically have? (A glass of wine or a beer counts as one drink.)

   A. One or two
   B. Three or four
   C. Five or six
   D. More than six

8. How often do you use marijuana?

   A. Daily or almost daily
   B. Four or five times a week
   C. Two or three times a week
   D. Once a week
   E. One to three times a month
   F. A few times a year
   G. Less often than once a year
   H. Not at all

9. How often do you use cocaine?

   A. Daily or almost daily
   B. Four or five times a week
   C. Two or three times a week
   D. Once a week
   E. One to three times a month
   F. A few times a year
   G. Less often than once a year
   H. Not at all

10. Have you ever used a nonprescription drug by injection?

   A. Yes
   B. No

11. What forms of contraception do you currently use, if any? (circle all that apply)

A. None
B. Birth control pills
C. Diaphragm
D. Foam or jelly
E. IUD (intrauterine device)
F. Condoms
G. Tubal ligation
H. Vasectomy
I. Rhythm method
J. Withdrawal
K. Douching
L. The intravaginal sponge
M. Other (please describe) _____

12. What is the *primary* method of contraception you rely on?

A. None
B. Birth control pills
C. Diaphragm
D. Foam or jelly
E. IUD (intrauterine device)
F. Condoms
G. Tubal ligation
H. Vasectomy
I. Rhythm method
J. Withdrawal
K. Douching
L. The intravaginal sponge
M. Other (please describe) _____

13. How often have you and your partner(s) used condoms during the past year?

A. All the time
B. Regularly (more than two-thirds of the time)
C. Occasionally

D. Infrequently (less than 10% of the time)
E. Never

PART III. SEXUAL BEHAVIOR

1. How old were you when you first had sexual intercourse?

_____

2. During the last 12 months, how many sexual partners have you had?

   A. None
   B. One
   C. Two or three
   D. Four or five
   E. Six to nine
   F. 10–14
   G. 15–19
   H. 20–24
   I. 25 or more

3. For each of the five years listed, please indicate by circling the appropriate numbers the number of sex partners you had.

Year			Number of Partners						
1986	0	1	2–3	4–5	6–9	10–14	15–19	20–24	25+
1985	0	1	2–3	4–5	6–9	10–14	15–19	20–24	25+
1984	0	1	2–3	4–5	6–9	10–14	15–19	20–24	25+
1983	0	1	2–3	4–5	6–9	10–14	15–19	20–24	25+
1982	0	1	2–3	4–5	6–9	10–14	15–19	20–24	25+

4. In the past year, have you participated in any of the following types of sexual activity? (circle answers)

   Self-masturbation to orgasm   Yes   No
   Manual stimulation by your partner to
     orgasm   Yes   No

Giving oral sex to your partner	Yes	No
Receiving oral sex from your partner	Yes	No
Vaginal intercourse	Yes	No
Anal intercourse	Yes	No

5. In the past year, what has been your average monthly frequency for each of the following types of sexual activity?

Self-masturbation to orgasm   _____ times per month

Manual stimulation by your
   partner to orgasm   _____ times per month

Giving oral sex to your
   partner   _____ times per month

Receiving oral sex from your
   partner   _____ times per month

Vaginal intercourse   _____ times per month

6. In the past year, what was your frequency of having anal intercourse? (circle one answer only)

   A. Daily or almost daily
   B. Four or five times a week
   C. Two or three times a week
   D. Once a week
   E. One to three times a month
   F. Once every two or three months
   G. One to three times during the year
   H. Not at all

7. [For men] Do you currently have any difficulties with (circle all that apply):

   A. Too little interest in sex
   B. Too much interest in sex

    C. Getting or keeping an erection
    D. Ejaculating too quickly
    E. Taking too long to ejaculate
    F. Being unable to ejaculate
    G. Pain during intercourse
    H. None of the above

8. [For women] Do you currently have any difficulties with (circle all that apply):

    A. Too little interest in sex
    B. Too much interest in sex
    C. Becoming sexually aroused
    D. Being unable to reach orgasm
    E. Taking too long to reach orgasm
    F. Reaching orgasm too quickly
    G. Pain during intercourse
    H. None of the above

9. With how many people have you ever had sexual relations?

    A. Your total number of male sex partners _____
    B. Your total number of female sex partners _____

10. If you are married, engaged, or living with someone, have you been completely faithful sexually to that person during the entire time of your relationship?

    A. Yes
    B. No

11. If you are married, engaged, or living with someone, do you think your partner has been completely faithful to you during the entire time of your relationship?

    A. Absolutely; I'm certain of this.
    B. Probably; I'm pretty sure, but not certain.

C. Possibly; I think so, but I'm not too sure.

D. Unlikely, but I don't know for a fact.

E. No.

12. Do you think that it is possible that you have been exposed to the AIDS virus in the past year?

A. Yes

B. No

C. Not sure

13. Do you think that there is any real risk of AIDS among heterosexuals who don't use intravenous drugs?

A. Yes

B. No

C. Not sure

14. Do you think that you can recognize someone who's infected with the AIDS virus?

A. Yes

B. No

C. Not sure

Would you like to make any comments about this questionnaire?

_____

_____

_____

_____

_____

_____

THANK YOU FOR YOUR PARTICIPATION IN THIS STUDY.

APPENDIX C
COMPULSORY PREMARITAL SCREENING FOR HIV: A TECHNICAL REANALYSIS OF THE HARVARD STUDY

In the October 2, 1987, issue of the *Journal of the American Medical Association,* a group of researchers from Harvard (the Harvard Study Group) published their analysis of the predicted effectiveness of a mandatory premarital HIV screening program in the United States. In Chapter 9, we indicated that while we agreed with the general framework of their analytic model, we disagreed with one key set of assumptions they used in their calculations. Specifically, we provided strong evidence from a variety of research reports that the Harvard Study Group's figures for the prevalence of HIV infection in the premarital population were far too low. To recap the issue here, we believe that rather than assuming a prevalence rate of 7 per 100,000 for all women applying for marriage licenses, a prevalence figure of 60 per 100,000 (drawn from the extensive military screening of female recruits and personnel) would be more accurate for females less than 35 years old. For males, we use three different prevalence rates instead of the Harvard team's figure of 70 per 100,000 for all males between the ages of 18 and 45. We apply a rate of 160 per 100,000 (also taken from the extensive military testing data) to 95% of the male population below age 45 (Group A below), on the assumption that these men are heterosexuals who do not use illicit drugs intravenously. For the remaining 5% of the population of male marriage license applicants under age 45 (Group B below), which we believe can be reasonably assumed to consist of homosexual, bisexual, and drug-using males, we apply a prevalence rate of 10% (10,000 per 100,000). For all other men and women—that is, women 35 and over, and men 45 and over, we use the same prevalence assumption as the Harvard Study Group, 7 per 100,000.

Applying these assumptions to the U.S. vital statistics data used by the Harvard researchers, we derive very different projections for the number of persons applying for marriage licenses who will be infected with the AIDS virus. Here are our computations:

			WOMEN		
Ages	*Number*		*Prevalence Rate Multiplier*		*Number Infected*
14–17	84,943	×	(.0006)	=	51
18–19	255,254	×	(.0006)	=	153
20–24	685,773	×	(.0006)	=	411
25–29	395,910	×	(.0006)	=	238
30–34	201,921	×	(.0006)	=	121
35–44	171,884	×	(.00007)	=	12
45–64	98,706	×	(.00007)	=	7
≥ 65	18,293	×	(.00007)	=	1
Subtotal					994

			MEN		
14–17	12,818				
	[A] 12,177	×	(.0016)	=	20
	[B] 641	×	(.10)	=	64
18–19	119,652				
	[A] 113,669	×	(.0016)	=	182
	[B] 5,983	×	(.10)	=	598

(MEN—*computations continued*)

20–24		632,089				
	[A]	600,485	×	(.0016)	=	961
	[B]	31,605	×	(.10)	=	3,161
25–29		477,761				
	[A]	453,873	×	(.0016)	=	726
	[B]	23,888	×	(.10)	=	2,388
30–34		258,802				
	[A]	245,861	×	(.0016)	=	393
	[B]	12,940	×	(.10)	=	1,294
35–44		228,931				
	[A]	217,485	×	(.0016)	=	348
	[B]	11,446	×	(.10)	=	1,145
≥45		182,631	×	(.00007)	=	13
	Subtotal					11,293

In addition to the above totals, the Harvard Study Group assumed that 60% of the couples applying for marriage licenses would have had sexual intercourse before screening and that among these couples, where one was HIV-infected, there would be a 10% transmission rate of the AIDS virus. (For purposes of this computation, it was assumed that HIV-infected persons only planned to marry persons who weren't infected.) Applying these same assumptions to the numbers we computed above, we find:

Additional # of HIV-infected men =
10% of 60% of 994 HIV-infected women

or

(.10) × (.60) × 994 = 59.6, rounded off to 60

Additional # of HIV-infected women =
10 percent of 60 percent of 11,293 HIV-infected men

or

(.10) × (.60) × 11,293 = 677.6, rounded off to 678

Adding the numbers of HIV-infected individuals computed from the prevalence figures to the numbers of persons predicted to be infected because of premarital transmission from an infected partner, we have:

     994 HIV-infected women
     678 women infected by transmission from their
            partners
 11,293 HIV-infected men
      60 men infected by transmission from their
            partners
  ———
 13,025 total infected individuals in the premarital
            population

To find out how many of these individuals will actually be detected in the premarital screening process, we use exactly the same assumptions used by the Harvard Study Group about the sensitivity and specificity of the ELISA and Western blot tests: ELISA screening results are based on an assumed sensitivity of 98.3% and an assumed specificity of 99.8%, while the comparable values for the Western blot test are 92% and 95% respectively. This gives the results shown in Table C.1, which can be summarized here by saying that out of 3,825,368 ELISA tests performed, with 12,802 Western blot tests for confirmation of ELISA positives, 11,778 cases of HIV infection will be correctly identified, 1,245 cases of infection will be missed, and 381 individuals will have false positive results.

Thus, by simply using prevalence assumptions that are much more accurately in tune with rates obtained by a variety of other researchers, we have reached conclusions quite different from those of the Harvard Study Group, whose model projected that only 1,219 infected persons would be correctly identified. Unless one feels that identifying almost 12,000

TABLE C.1

Projected ELISA and Western Blot Test Performance in First Year of a Premarital Screening Program, Based on Modified Prevalence Assumptions

| ELISA Results | NUMBER OF PERSONS | | |
	HIV-Infected	Not HIV-Infected	Total
Positive (+)	12,802	7,625	20,427
Negative (−)	221	3,804,720	3,804,941
Total	13,023[a]	3,812,345	3,825,368
Western Blot Results			
ELISA+, WB+	11,778	381	12,159
ELISA+, WB−	1,024	7,244	8,268
Not tested (ELISA−)	221	3,804,720	3,804,941
Total	13,023[a]	3,812,345	3,825,368

[a]The minor discrepancy between this figure and the total mentioned above in the text (13,025) is due to rounding off decimals.

cases of HIV infection in the first year of a mandatory premarital screening program is not a worthwhile accomplishment, it would seem that such a program has far more efficiency and utility than the Harvard group ascribes to it. This conclusion becomes even more vivid when it is realized that a substantial number of HIV infections in babies may be averted by mandatory premarital testing. In fact, using the basic model specified by the Harvard Study Group but substituting our more realistic figures for the number of seropositive women who would be detected in a compulsory premarital screening program, we estimate that approximately 5,000 infected births might be prevented by one year of screening. Needless to say, as the prevalence of infection rises in the general population, this number would rise proportionately.

NOTES

Key to abbreviations:

CDC   U.S. Centers for Disease Control
JAMA   *Journal of the American Medical Association*
MMWR   *Morbidity and Mortality Weekly Report*
NEJM   *New England Journal of Medicine*

A citation such as "n. 1.3" means that the work in question has already been cited and that the full reference can be found in note 3 of the notes to Chapter 1.

CHAPTER 1

1. S. J. Gould, "The Terrifying Normalcy of AIDS," *New York Times Magazine*, April 19, 1987, pp. 32–33.
2. For example, the CDC reported in 1986 that "the relative proportion of AIDS cases among most risk groups has remained stable" (*MMWR* 35:17–21, 1986). Dr. Harold Jaffe, chief AIDS epidemiologist at the CDC, was quoted during the Third International Conference on AIDS in mid-1987 as stating that "no explosive growth of acquired immune deficiency syndrome was occurring among heterosexuals" (reported by L. K. Altman, "AIDS Expert Sees No Sign of Heterosexual Outbreak," *New York Times*, June 5, 1987, p. A17). This remark may have been true in a limited sense—the actual number of cases of AIDS, the disease, in heterosexuals may not have been exploding—but given the long latency period between the time of infection and the appearance of the disease itself, the statement did not ad-

dress what was actually happening in terms of patterns of infection. Another news story in *The New York Times,* under the headline "AIDS Spread Seen in Same Patterns" (October 11, 1987, p. 44), quoted the New York City Health Department's director of AIDS research as saying "nothing has changed" in the pattern of infection with the AIDS virus, although a careful reading of the story shows otherwise.

3. The original estimate is given in Coolfont Report: A PHS plan for prevention and control of AIDS and the AIDS virus, *Public Health Reports* 101: 341–48, 1986; and Institute of Medicine/ National Academy of Sciences, *Confronting AIDS: Directions for Public Health, Health Care, and Research* (Washington, D.C.: National Academy Press, 1986). In December 1987, health officials reportedly informed the White House that "they saw no reason to revise their previous estimate . . . that 1 to 1.5 million Americans have already been infected with the AIDS virus" (P. M. Boffey, "U.S. to Test for AIDS in 30 Cities; Household Sampling Put Off," *New York Times,* December 3, 1987, p. A20).

4. A number of authorities have estimated that there are 50 to 100 people infected with the AIDS virus for every actual case of AIDS. See, for example, R. R. Redfield and D. S. Burke, Shadow on the land: The epidemiology of HIV infection, *Viral Immunology* 1 (1): 69–81, 1987; and H. Mahler, opening speech to the Second International Conference on AIDS, Paris, June 23–25, 1986. (Mahler, who is director of the World Health Organization, noted, "AIDS, the syndrome, is only the tip of the iceberg; for every AIDS case there are three to five cases of the less severe AIDS-related complex and anything between 50 and 100 silent carriers.") Since the cumulative total of cases of AIDS in the United States as of late 1987 was approximately 45,000, we can calculate (using the midpoint figure of 75 as our multiplier) that the pool of infected people was approximately 3,375,000 as of that time.

5. T. A. Bell and K. Hein, "Adolescents and Sexually Transmitted Diseases," in K. K. Holmes et al., eds., *Sexually Transmitted Diseases* (New York: McGraw-Hill, 1984), pp. 73–84. In a different chapter of the same book ("Prevention of Sexually Transmitted Diseases" pp. 973–91) J. W. Curran notes, "The most dependable determinant of STD [sexually transmitted disease] occurrence is age. In the United States, teenagers and young adults account for

an increasing share of reported STDs" (p. 977). As partial documentation of this observation, Curran points out that in 1980, 83% of gonorrhea cases were reported among persons 15 to 29 years of age. In addition, cases of AIDS among U.S. teenagers rose by 54% in the first eleven months of 1987 (J. Johnson, "Nation Found Lacking on Infant AIDS Threat," *New York Times*, December 14, 1987, p. A20).

6. *Surgeon General's Report on Acquired Immune Deficiency Syndrome* (Washington, D.C.: U.S. Department of Health and Human Services, 1986).

7. CDC, Positive HTLV-III/LAV antibody results for sexually active female members of social/sexual clubs—Minnesota, *MMWR* 35: 697–99, 1986.

8. We base this observation on our own unpublished sex research data, which has been gathered over more than three decades. Exactly the same point is made in B. B. Dan, Sex and the singles' whirl: the quantum dynamics of hepatitis B, *JAMA* 256: 1344, 1986.

9. P. Piot et al., Acquired immunodeficiency syndrome in an heterosexual population in Zaire, *Lancet* 2: 65–69, 1984; N. Clumeck et al., Seroepidemiological studies of HTLV-III antibody prevalence among selected groups of heterosexual Africans, *JAMA* 254: 2599–2602, 1985; T. C. Quinn et al., AIDS in Africa: An epidemiologic paradigm, *Science* 234: 955–63, 1986; R. J. Biggar, The AIDS problem in Africa, *Lancet* 1: 79–82, 1986; J. K. Kreiss et al., AIDS virus infection in Nairobi prostitutes, *NEJM* 314: 414–18, 1986.

10. W. B. Johnson (Cornell Medical College), personal communication on epidemiology of AIDS and HIV infection in Haiti, July 11, 1986, cited in L. Liskin and B. Blackburn, AIDS—A public health crisis, *Population Reports*, series L, no. 6, July–August 1986.

11. J. Palca, AIDS virus at the centre, *Nature* 319: 170, 1987; Richard Selzer, "A Mask on the Face of Death," *Life*, August 1987, pp. 59–64.

12. T. A. Peterman and J. W. Curran, Sexual transmission of human immunodeficiency virus, *JAMA* 256: 2222, 1986.

13. Institute of Medicine/National Academy of Sciences, n. 1.3; Liskin and Blackburn, n. 1.10.

14. Mahler, n. 1.14.

15. See, for example, W. King, "Doctors Cite Stigma of AIDS in

Declining to Report Cases," *New York Times,* May 27, 1986, p. A1; "MD Left AIDS Off Patient's Death Certificate," *American Medical News,* August 14, 1987, p. 35; "Failure to List AIDS on Death Certificates Criticized," *American Medical News,* October 2, 1987, p. 42; A. H. Hardy et al., Review of death certificates to assess completeness of AIDS case reporting, *Public Health Reports* 102: 386–91, 1987; T. Kircher and R. E. Anderson, Cause of death—Proper completion of the death certificate, *JAMA* 258: 349–52, 1987.

16. CDC, Revision of the CDC surveillance case definition for acquired immunodeficiency syndrome, *MMWR* 36, supplement 1S, 1987. The new definition, announced on August 14, 1987, was to be applied to actual case reporting beginning September 1, 1987.

17. CDC, Revision of the case definition of acquired immunodeficiency syndrome for national reporting—United States, *MMWR* 34: 373–75, 1985.

18. Coolfont Report, n. 1.3.

19. Ibid. The report itself notes that "the empirical model [used for calculating future trends] may underestimate by at least 20 percent the serious morbidity and mortality attributable to AIDS, because of underreporting or underascertainment of cases."

CHAPTER 2

1. "Youth's Puzzling Death in '69 May Be Early U.S. AIDS Case," *New York Times,* October 26, 1987, p. B9; G. Kolata, "Boy's 1969 Death Suggests AIDS Invaded U.S. Several Times," *New York Times,* October 28, 1987, p. A15.

2. M. D. Daniel et al., Isolation of T-cell tropic HTLV-III-like retrovirus from macaques, *Science* 228: 1201–4, 1985; P. J. Kanki, J. Alroy, and M. Essex, Isolation of T-lymphotropic retrovirus related to HTLV-III/LAV from wild-caught African green monkeys, *Science* 230: 951–54, 1985; M. Murphey-Corb et al., Isolation of an HTLV-III-related retrovirus from macaques with simian AIDS and its possible origin in asymptomatic mangabeys, *Nature* 321: 435–37, 1986; N. L. Letvin and R. D. Desrosiers, Animal models for AIDS and their use for vaccine and drug development (Washington, D.C.: Committee on a National Strategy for AIDS, 1986), background paper.

3. CDC, *Pneumocystis* pneumonia—Los Angeles, *MMWR* 30: 250–52, 1981; A. Friedman-Kien et al., Kaposi's sarcoma and *Pneumocystis* pneumonia among homosexual men in New York City and California, *MMWR* 30: 305–8, 1981.

4. S. F. Lyons et al., Lack of evidence of HTLV-III endemicity in southern Africa, *NEJM* 312: 1257–58, 1985; R. Sher et al., Sero-epidemiology of human immunodeficiency virus in Africa from 1970 to 1974, *NEJM* 317: 450–51, 1987.

5. The Russians have finally retracted this accusation. See "Soviet Disavows Charges That U.S. Created AIDS," *New York Times*, November 5, 1987, p. A31.

6. D. L. Breo, "AMA AIDS Expert's Grim Message," *American Medical News*, December 5, 1986, p. 3; M. Chase, "AIDS Conferees Share New Hopes, New Fears in Battling the Disease," *Wall Street Journal*, April 13, 1987, p. 25; L. K. Altman, "AIDS Virus: Always Fatal?" *New York Times*, September 8, 1987, p. C1.

7. D. D. Ho, R. J. Pomerantz, and J. C. Kaplan, Pathogenesis of infection with human immunodeficiency virus, *NEJM* 317: 278–86, 1987.

8. C. A. Raymond, Evidence mounts that other infections may trigger AIDS virus replication, *JAMA* 257: 2875, 1987; G. Nabel and D. Baltimore, An inducible transcription factor activates expression of human immunodeficiency virus in T cells, *Nature* 326: 711–13, 1987; J. J. Potterat, Does syphilis facilitate sexual transmission of HIV? [letter], *JAMA* 258: 473, 1987; T. C. Quinn et al., Serologic and immunologic studies in patients with AIDS in North America and Africa, *JAMA* 257: 2617–21, 1987.

9. Ho, Pomerantz, and Kaplan, n. 2.7.

10. J. E. Groopman and J. Gurley, "Biology of HIV Infection," in *Information on AIDS for the Practicing Physician*, vol. 2 (Chicago: American Medical Association, 1987), pp. 17–23 (quoted phrase appears on p. 19).

11. Peterman and Curran, n. 1.12; R. M. Grant, J. A. Wiley, and W. Winkelstein, Infectivity of the human immunodeficiency virus: Estimates from a prospective study of homosexual men, *Journal of Infectious Diseases* 156: 189–93, 1987; J. J. Goedert, What is safe sex? *NEJM* 316: 1339–42, 1987; N. Padian et al., Male-to-female transmission of human immunodeficiency virus, *JAMA* 258: 788–90, 1987.

12. D. R. Bolling, Prevalence, goals, and complications of heterosex-

ual anal intercourse in a gynecologic population, *Journal of Reproductive Medicine* 19: 120–24, 1977; J. Agnew, Hazards associated with anal erotic activity, *Archives of Sexual Behavior* 15: 307–14, 1986; Institute of Medicine/National Academy of Sciences, n. 1.3; Peterman and Curran, n. 1.12.

13. R. R. Redfield et al., Heterosexually acquired HTLV-III/LAV disease (AIDS-related complex and AIDS), *JAMA* 254: 2094–96, 1985; Peterman and Curran, n. 1.12; L. H. Calabrese and K. V. Gopalakrishna, Transmission of HTLV-III infection from man to woman to man, *NEJM* 314: 987, 1986; B. R. Saltzman et al., HTLV-III/LAV infection and immunodeficiency in heterosexual partners of AIDS patients, *Abstracts of the Second International Conference on AIDS* (1986), p. 125; N. Padian, Heterosexual transmission of acquired immunodeficiency syndrome: International perspectives and national projections, *Reviews of Infectious Diseases* 9: 947–60, 1987; M. Chamberland and T. Dondero, Heterosexually acquired infection with human immunodeficiency virus (HIV), *Annals of Internal Medicine* 107: 763–66, 1987.

14. M. A. Fischl et al., Evaluation of heterosexual partners, children, and household contacts of adults with AIDS, *JAMA* 257: 640–44, 1987. These researchers noted that 14 of 28 female spouses of men with AIDS showed evidence of infection with the AIDS virus; however, "anal intercourse was not a common practice and did not appear to play a significant role in the heterosexual transmission of HTLV-III/LAV" (pp. 643–44).

15. Padian et al., n. 2.11.

16. This level of risk is supported by a computer model reported by A. M. Salzberg et al., Male-to-female transmission of HIV, *JAMA* 258: 3386, 1987.

17. D. D. Ho et al., HTLV-III in semen and blood of a healthy homosexual man, *Science* 226: 451–53, 1984; D. Zagury et al., HTLV-III in cells cultured from semen of two patients with AIDS, *Science* 226: 449–51, 1984.

18. C. B. Wofsy et al., Isolation of AIDS-associated retrovirus from genital secretions of women with antibodies to the virus, *Lancet* 1: 527–29, 1986; D. W. Archibald et al., Antibodies to HIV in cervical secretions from women at risk of AIDS, *Journal of Infectious Diseases* 156: 240–41, 1987.

19. Liskin and Blackburn, n. 1.10.

20. *Surgeon General's Report,* n. 1.6.

21. W. Winkelstein et al., Sexual practices and risk of infection by the human immunodeficiency virus, *JAMA* 257: 321–25, 1987.
22. Padian et al., n. 2.11.
23. Fischl et al., n. 2.14.
24. For example, cases of pharyngeal gonorrhea or syphilis are well known. The pharynx is infected in about 5% of heterosexual men and 10% to 20% of heterosexual women with gonorrhea. The classical primary syphilis chancre occurs with some frequency on the lips and tongue or in other areas inside the mouth, including the tonsils. Cases of chlamydial pharyngitis in both men and women have been reported. Genital herpes is, of course, a common result of oral-genital contact. And hepatitis B, which has the highest prevalence in homosexual men, can be transmitted by oral-genital sex as well as anal and vaginal intercourse. But even rarer STDs, such as chancroid (caused by *Haemophilus ducreyi*) and donovanosis (caused by *Calymmatobacterium granulomatis*), have been reported to be transmitted by oral sex— see, for example, B. R. Garg et al., Donovanosis (granuloma inguinale) of the oral cavity, *British Journal of Venereal Disease* 51: 136, 1975.
25. J. E. Groopman et al., HTLV-III in saliva of people with AIDS-related complex and healthy homosexual men at risk for AIDS, *Science* 226: 447–49, 1984; D. D. Ho et al., Infrequency of isolation of HTLV-III virus from saliva in AIDS, *NEJM* 313: 1606, 1985.
26. See, for example, the discussions in Institute of Medicine/National Academy of Sciences, n. 1.3; and *Surgeon General's Report*, n. 1.6.
27. T. J. Spira, et al., Prevalence of antibody to lymphadenopathy-associated virus among drug detoxification patients in New York, *NEJM* 311: 467–69, 1984; D. E. Craven, L. M. Kunches, and J. E. Groopman, Prevalence of antibodies to HTLV-III in parenteral drug abusers attending a methadone clinic (presented at the First International Conference on AIDS, Atlanta, April 14–17, 1985); R. D'Aquila et al., Prevalence of HTLV-III infection among New Haven, Connecticut parenteral drug abusers in 1982–1983, *NEJM* 314: 117–18, 1986; D. I. Macdonald, IV drugs and AIDS—San Francisco, *JAMA* 258: 2642, 1987.
28. H. G. Klein and H. J. Alter, "Blood Transfusion and AIDS," in *Information on AIDS*, n. 2.10, pp. 7–10.

29. Although the heating of clotting factors has greatly reduced the risk of infection with HIV among hemophiliacs, reports of cases of seroconversion despite the exclusive use of heated clotting factors have continued to appear. See, for example, G. C. White, HTLV-III seroconversion associated with heat-treated factor VIII concentrate, *Lancet* 1: 611–12, 1986; G. Mariani et al., Heated clotting factors and seroconversion for human immunodeficiency virus in three hemophiliac patients, *Annals of Internal Medicine* 107: 113, 1987; CDC, Survey of non-U.S. hemophilia treatment centers for HIV seroconversions following therapy with heat-treated factor concentrates, *MMWR* 36: 121–24, 1987.

30. Klein and Alter, n. 2.28, p. 8.

31. Ibid.

32. Liskin and Blackburn, n. 1.10.

33. CDC, Update: Acquired immunodeficiency syndrome—United States, *MMWR* 35: 757–66, 1986.

34. G. B. Scott et al., Mothers of infants with acquired immunodeficiency syndrome: Evidence for both symptomatic and asymptomatic carriers, *JAMA* 253: 363–66, 1985; W. A. Ledger, "AIDS and the Obstetrician/Gynecologist: Commentary," in *Information on AIDS*, n. 2.10, pp. 5–6; J. Q. Mok et al., Infants born to mothers seropositive for human immunodeficiency virus, *Lancet* 1: 1164–67, 1987.

35. L. Thiry et al., Isolation of AIDS virus from cell-free breast milk of three healthy virus carriers, *Lancet* 2: 891–92, 1985.

36. J. B. Ziegler et al., Postnatal transmission of AIDS-associated retrovirus from mother to infant, *Lancet* 1: 896–98, 1985.

37. For instance, in one report, none of 101 medical workers with heavy occupational exposure to AIDS patients tested seropositive (A. Moss et al., Risk of seroconversion for acquired immunodeficiency syndrome in San Francisco health workers, *Journal of Occupational Medicine* 28: 821–24, 1986). In another report, on 361 health care and clinical laboratory workers, 3 of 44 workers with needlestick injuries were reported to be seropositive (S. H. Weiss, HTLV-III infection among health-care workers, *JAMA* 254: 2089–93, 1985). In one other study, only 2 of 320 health care workers who had needlestick exposure to blood or other body fluids from AIDS patients tested positive for HIV antibodies (E. McCray, Occupational risk of acquired im-

munodeficiency syndrome among health care workers, *NEJM* 314: 1127–32, 1986). Some exceptions (the relatively rare cases where needlestick injury resulted in HIV infection) were reported in the following: Needlestick transmission of HTLV-III from a patient infected in Africa, *Lancet* 2: 1376–77, 1984; R. L. Stricof and D. L. Morse, HTLV-III seroconversion following a deep intramuscular needlestick injury, *NEJM* 314: 1115, 1986; E. Oksenhendler et al., HIV infection with seroconversion after a superficial needlestick injury to the finger, *NEJM* 315: 582, 1986; and C. Neisson-Vernant et al., Needlestick HIV seroconversion in a nurse, *Lancet* 2: 814, 1986. At San Francisco General Hospital, which is widely regarded as the nation's leading AIDS hospital, some personnel became very upset upon learning in October 1987 that a health care worker there seroconverted after a needlestick injury. The chief of orthopedic surgery at the hospital, Dr. Lorraine Day, voiced her strong reaction as follows: "We're told that one of our hospital workers seroconverted. The word seroconversion makes it sound like they got religion or something. Let's be more honest. Let's say the worker has contracted a terminal illness and will die." Dr. Day went on to say that many of the hospital's AIDS experts privately suspect that everyone who becomes infected with the AIDS virus will eventually develop full-blown AIDS and die (S. Staver, "Orthopod Urges HIV Testing," *American Medical News,* December 4, 1987, pp. 1, 36–37; quoted material appears on p. 37).

38. CDC, Update: Human immunodeficiency virus infections in health-care workers exposed to blood of infected patients, *MMWR* 36: 285–89, 1987.

39. J. L. Baker et al., Unsuspected human immunodeficiency virus in critically ill emergency patients, *JAMA* 257: 2609–11, 1987.

CHAPTER 3

1. See, for example, D. A. Cooper et al., Acute AIDS retrovirus infection: Definition of a clinical illness associated with seroconversion, *Lancet* 1: 547–50, 1985; C. A. Carne et al., Acute encephalopathy coincident with seroconversion for anti-HTLV-III, *Lancet* 2: 1206–8, 1985; J. Tucker et al., HTLV-III infection associated with glandular-fever-like illness in a haemophiliac, *Lancet* 1: 585, 1985; R. Lindskov et al., Acute HTLV-III infection

with roseola-like rash, *Lancet* 1: 447, 1986; H. A. Kessler et al., Diagnosis of human immunodeficiency virus infection in seronegative homosexuals presenting with an acute viral syndrome, *JAMA* 258: 1196–99, 1987.

2. R. M. Levy, D. E. Bedesen, and M. L. Rosenblum, Neurological manifestations of the acquired immunodeficiency syndrome (AIDS): Experience at UCSF and review of the literature, *Journal of Neurosurgery* 62: 475–95, 1985; H. Hollander and J. A. Levy, Neurologic abnormalities and recovery of human immunodeficiency virus from cerebrospinal fluid, *Annals of Internal Medicine* 106: 692–95, 1987; D. H. Gabuzda and M. S. Hirsch, Neurologic manifestations of infection with human immunodeficiency virus, *Annals of Internal Medicine* 107: 383–91, 1987.

3. Liskin and Blackburn, n. 1.10; Institute of Medicine/National Academy of Sciences, n. 1.3.

4. Ho, Pomerantz, and Kaplan, n. 2.7, p. 283.

5. R. A. Weiss et al., Variable and conserved neutralization antigens of human immunodeficiency virus, *Nature* 324: 572–75, 1986; A. Ranki et al., Characterization of the latent period and the development of neutralizing antibodies in early sexually transmitted HIV infection [abstract], in *Third International Conference on Acquired Immunodeficiency Syndrome (AIDS)* (Washington, D.C.: U.S. Department of Health and Human Services, 1987), p. 30; S. Koenig and Z. F. Rosenberg, Immunology of infection with the human immunodeficiency virus (HIV), *Annals of Internal Medicine* 107: 409–12, 1987.

6. M. Melbye et al., Long-term seropositivity for human T-lymphotropic virus type III in homosexual men without the acquired immunodeficiency syndrome: Development of immunologic and clinical abnormalities, *Annals of Internal Medicine* 104: 496–500, 1986.

7. B. F. Polk et al., Predictors of the acquired immunodeficiency syndrome developing in a cohort of seropositive homosexual men, *NEJM* 316: 61–66, 1987; J. J. Goedert et al., Effect of T4 count and cofactors on the incidence of AIDS in homosexual men infected with human immunodeficiency virus, *JAMA* 257: 331–34, 1987.

8. Ibid.

9. Quinn et al., n. 2.8.

10. M. Troye-Blomberg et al., Regulation of the immune response in *Plasmodium falciparum* malaria, *Clinical and Experimental Immunology* 58: 380–87, 1984; R. G. Marlink, Africa and the biology of human immunodeficiency virus, *JAMA* 257: 2632–33, 1987.

11. Quinn et al., n. 2.8; Padian, n. 2.13; Selzer, n. 1.11. In addition, many experts think that heterosexually transmitted HIV infection is very common in Africa and Haiti because of the high prevalence in those areas of ulcerations or sores on the genitals in both sexes, which may make it easier for the virus to enter the body during penile-vaginal intercourse. Another way in which cofactors may operate is this: if a man has gonorrhea (or a similar STD), he will have more white blood cells in his semen (due to the infection), which means that there will probably be more AIDS virus in his semen than he would otherwise have.

12. Groopman and Gurley, n. 2.10; C. Bohan et al., Transactivation of human immunodeficiency virus by herpes virus [abstract], in *Third International Conference*, n. 3.5, p. 14.

13. Nabel and Baltimore, n. 2.8.

14. Institute of Medicine/National Academy of Sciences, n. 1.3, p. 65.

15. D. B. Fishbein et al., Unexplained lymphadenopathy in homosexual men, *JAMA* 254: 930–35, 1985; U. Mathur-Wagh, D. Mildvan, and R. T. Senie, Follow-up at 4½ years on homosexual men with generalized lymphadenopathy, *NEJM* 313: 1542–43, 1985; J. E. Kaplan et al., Lymphadenopathy syndrome in homosexual men, *JAMA* 257: 335–37, 1987.

16. R. S. Holzman, C. M. Walsh, and S. Karpatkin, Risk for the acquired immunodeficiency syndrome among thrombocytopenic and nonthrombocytopenic homosexual men seropositive for the human immunodeficiency virus, *Annals of Internal Medicine* 106: 383–86, 1987.

17. B. Johnstone, German survey's gloomy outlook, *Nature* 324: 199, 1986. In this report of a paper presented in *Deutsche Medizinische Wochenschrift* in 1986, computer forecasts based on previous trends seen in 543 patients, who were largely the sexual partners of the first AIDS victims to die in Frankfurt, project that 50% of HIV antibody carriers will progress to full-scale AIDS within five years of their first exposure and 75% will have AIDS within seven years.

18. B. Lambert, "AIDS Forecasts Are Grim—and Disparate," *New York Times,* October 25, 1987, section 4, p. 24. See also the comment by Dr. Lorraine Day in n. 2.37.
19. R. C. Gallo et al., Frequent detection and isolation of cytopathic retroviruses (HTLV-III) from patients with AIDS and at risk for AIDS, *Science* 224: 500–502, 1984; J. A. Levy and J. Shimabukuro, Recovery of AIDS-associated retroviruses from patients with AIDS, AIDS-related conditions, and clinically healthy individuals, *Journal of Infectious Diseases* 152: 734–38, 1985; B. A. Michaelis and J. A. Levy, Recovery of human immunodeficiency virus from serum, *JAMA* 257: 1327, 1987.
20. J. J. Goedert, Testing for human immunodeficiency virus, *Annals of Internal Medicine* 105: 609–10, 1986; J. W. Ward et al., Laboratory and epidemiologic evaluation of an enzyme immunoassay for antibodies to HTLV-III, *JAMA* 256: 357–61, 1986; A. M. Courouce, Evaluation of eight ELISA kits for the detection of anti-LAV/HTLV-III antibodies, *Lancet* 1: 1152–53, 1986; G. Ujhelyi et al., Studies of the sensitivity and reproducibility of commercial kits to detect antibodies to human immunodeficiency virus, *Transfusion* 27: 210–12, 1987.
21. Ward et al, n. 3.20.
22. An example of the imprecision of the Western blot test can be found in a 1985 study in which 10 of 69 AIDS patients were negative on both ELISA and Western blot testing (J. R. Carlson et al., AIDS serology testing in low- and high-risk groups, *JAMA* 253: 3405–8, 1985). False positives have also been reported with Western blot testing (see, for example, D. S. Burke and R. R. Redfield, False-positive Western blot tests for antibodies to HTLV-III, *JAMA* 256: 347, 1986; and G. Biberfeld et al., Blood donor sera with false-positive Western blot reactions to human immunodeficiency virus, *Lancet* 2: 289–90, 1986).
23. S. Z. Salahuddin et al., HTLV-III in symptom-free seronegative persons, *Lancet* 2: 1418, 1984; J. P. Phair, Human immunodeficiency virus antigenemia, *JAMA* 258: 1218, 1987; A. Ranki et al., Long latency precedes overt seroconversion in sexually transmitted human-immunodeficiency-virus infections, *Lancet* 2: 589–93, 1987.
24. D. D. Ho et al., Primary human T-lymphotropic virus type III infection, *Annals of Internal Medicine* 103: 880–83, 1985; Institute of Medicine/National Academy of Sciences, n. 1.3; A. J. Saah,

"Serologic Tests for Human Immunodeficiency Virus (HIV)," in *Information on AIDS*, n. 2.10, pp. 11–16.

25. Institute of Medicine/National Academy of Sciences, n. 1.3, p. 114.

26. Consensus Conference, The impact of routine HTLV-III antibody testing of blood and plasma donors on public health, *JAMA* 256: 1778–83, 1986 (quoted material appears on p. 1780).

27. C. Levine and R. Bayer, Screening blood: Public health and medical uncertainty, *Hastings Center Report,* special supplement, August 1985, pp. 8–11; R. Shilts, *And the Band Played On: Politics, People, and the AIDS Epidemic* (New York: St. Martin's Press, 1987), pp. 541–42, 552.

28. Saah, n. 3.24; Phair, n. 3.23; Kessler, n. 3.1.

CHAPTER 4

1. M. J. Alter et al., Hepatitis B virus transmission between heterosexuals, *JAMA* 256: 1307–10, 1986.

2. M. T. Schreeder et al., Hepatitis B in homosexual men: Prevalence of infection and factors related to transmission, *Journal of Infectious Diseases* 146: 7–15, 1982; S. M. Lemon, "Viral Hepatitis," in Holmes et al., n. 1.5, pp. 479–96.

3. Alter et al., n. 4.1, p. 1309.

4. It is interesting to see that an almost identical percentage of homosexual and bisexual men participating in a large multicenter study that involved HIV antibody testing declined to receive information on their test results. A report on the study by D. Lyter et al. (*Public Health Reports* 102: 468–74, 1987, cited in *JAMA* 258: 2349, 1987) noted that only 1,109 out of 2,047 homosexual and bisexual men (54%) chose to receive their HIV antibody test results. Of those men who didn't wish to know their results and responded to a questionnaire listing their reasons for not wanting to know, 16% said they didn't believe the HIV antibody test was predictive of developing AIDS, 18% believed the test was inaccurate, and others were worried about their emotional reaction to a positive test result.

5. For example, the Institute of Medicine/National Academy of Sciences report (n. 1.3, p. 9) notes, "Over the next 5 to 10 years there will be substantially more cases of HIV infection in the heterosexual population." The *Surgeon General's Report* (n. 1.6)

concurs, pointing out, "Heterosexual transmission is expected to account for an increasing proportion of those who become infected with the AIDS virus in the future." See also D. F. Echenberg, A new strategy to prevent the spread of AIDS among heterosexuals, *JAMA* 254: 2129–30, 1985; M. E. Guinan and A. Hardy, Epidemiology of AIDS in women in the United States—1981–1986, *JAMA* 257: 2039–42, 1987; E. E. Schoenbaum and M. H. Alderman, Antibody to the human immunodeficiency virus in New York City, *Annals of Internal Medicine* 107: 599, 1987; and Padian, n. 2.13.

6. I. L. Reiss et al., "Research on Heterosexual Relationships," in R. Green and J. Weiner, eds., *Methodology in Sex Research* (Rockville, Md.: U.S. Department of Health and Human Services, #ADM 80-766, 1980), pp. 1–57; W. H. Masters, V. E. Johnson, and R. C. Kolodny, "Sex Research: An Overview," in *Human Sexuality,* 2d ed. (Boston: Little, Brown, 1985), pp. 24–45.

7. *Surgeon General's Report,* n. 1.6; D. P. Francis and J. Chin, The prevention of acquired immunodeficiency syndrome in the United States, *JAMA* 257: 1357–66, 1987; Goedert, n. 2.11.

CHAPTER 5

1. Shilts, n. 3.27, pp. 220–26, 343–48, 432–35.
2. CDC, Human immunodeficiency virus infection in transfusion recipients and their family members, *MMWR* 36: 137–40, 1987. Such official reassurances repeatedly find their way into the press. For example, "Experts say blood supplies pose virtually no risk of infection since blood donations are now screened for contamination with the AIDS virus" (H. Stout, "40% of Americans Fear They Will Contract AIDS, A Poll Indicates," *New York Times,* November 29, 1987, p. 26).
3. Goedert, n. 3.20.
4. S. H. Weiss et al., Screening test for HTLV-III (AIDS agent) antibodies, *JAMA* 253: 221–25, 1985.
5. Carlson et al., n. 3.22.
6. A. J. Saah et al., Detection of early antibodies in human immunodeficiency virus infection by enzyme-linked immunosorbent assay, Western blot, and radioimmunoprecipitation, *Journal of Clinical Microbiology* 25: 1605–10, 1987. Saah and his colleagues noted that among a group of 106 Western-blot-confirmed sero-

converters in the Multicenter AIDS Cohort Study, 19 showed little or no reactivity to gp41 (one of the envelope antigens of HIV) at their six-month visit. These researchers observed, "Unless individuals who are seroconverting to HIV voluntarily refrain from donating blood or plasma, it seems highly likely that such contaminated blood would be misidentified, to various degrees, by the currently licensed kits" (p. 1609).

7. H. W. Reesink et al., Evaluation of six enzyme immunoassays for antibody against human immunodeficiency virus, *Lancet* 2: 483–86, 1986; Courouce et al., n. 3.20; G. Fust et al., Traps of HIV serology: Independent changes in sensitivity and specificity of ELISA kits, in *Third International Conference*, n. 3.5, p. 49; Ujhelyi et al., n. 3.20.

8. M. E. Lunz et al., The impact of quality of the laboratory staff on the accuracy of laboratory results, *JAMA* 258: 361–63, 1987. Problems with testing for HIV antibodies in some ways parallel difficulties in laboratory performance that have already been encountered in testing urine samples for illicit drugs. Some of these problems are discussed in E. J. Imwinkelried, False positive: Shoddy drug testing is jeopardizing the jobs of millions, *The Sciences* 27 (5): 23–28, 1987. Another paper on drug testing notes that many laboratory directors insist on doing a confirmatory second procedure "to ensure that there had been no administrative errors, such as a mix-up of samples" (D. W. Hoyt et al., Drug testing in the workplace—Are methods legally defensible? *JAMA* 258: 504–9, 1987; quote appears on p. 507). Likewise, in a recent book, Dr. John A. J. Barbara notes that "in a busy transfusion center" all sorts of mistakes can happen (J. C. Petricciani et al., eds., *AIDS: The Safety of Blood and Blood Products* [New York: WHO/John Wiley, 1987], pp. 166–67). Despite such widespread recognition of testing mix-ups and errors in even the best laboratories, virtually no attention has been paid to this problem in regard to mistakenly certifying HIV-infected blood as "antibody-free" and then allowing it to be used for transfusions.

9. D. B. Barnes, New questions about AIDS test accuracy, *Science* 238: 884–85, 1987.

10. T. F. Zuck, Greetings—A final look back with comments about a policy of zero-risk blood supply, *Transfusion* 27: 447–48, 1987.

11. Ranki et al., n. 3.23. In this study, which utilized retrospective testing of blood samples previously collected at three- to six-

month intervals from a group of homosexual men who were subsequently found to have become seropositive, it was reported that seroconversion took seven or eight months in 5 out of 9 men, while 2 out of the 9 men took thirteen or fourteen months to seroconvert. While this extraordinary finding has yet to be verified, its implications are particularly distressing since it suggests that cases in which there is a prolonged interval of infectivity before an ELISA-measurable antibody response occurs may be more widespread than has been thought.

12. Ho et al., n. 3.24; CDC, Transfusion-associated human T-lymphotropic virus type III/lymphadenopathy-associated virus from a seronegative donor—Colorado, *MMWR* 35: 389–91, 1986.

13. According to W. E. Kline et al. (Hepatitis B core antibody [anti-HBc] in blood donors in the United States: Implications for surrogate testing programs, *Transfusion* 27: 99–102, 1987), the American Red Cross collected approximately 6.1 million units of blood in the most recent year for which data were available (July 1, 1984, to June 30, 1985), and this represented half of the nation's blood supply. The average Red Cross donor gave blood 1.5 times per year. Thus, if the total number of units of blood donated in the U.S. was approximately 12 million, representing donations by some 8 million different donors, and the 1984 U.S. population for the age groups 18 to 64 was approximately 145 million (U.S. Bureau of the Census, *Statistical Abstract of the United States: 1986,* 106th ed. [Washington, D.C.: Government Printing Office, 1985], p. xvii), it can be estimated that approximately 5.5% of the American adult population under age 65 serve as blood donors in any given year. This means that our assumption of a 4% blood donor rate among persons with new cases of HIV infection who are neither homosexual or bisexual males nor IV drug users is a conservative one. Along the same lines, it is relevant to note that a blood bank in the San Francisco area conducting a look-back program found that of the approximately 2,500 patients with AIDS reported in their vicinity as of August 1986, 139 (5.5%) had donated blood at one blood bank since 1977; between 1977 and 1984, these 139 patients with AIDS had donated blood to over 950 people (M. Busch, S. Sampson, and H. Perkins, Is look-back doing the job? [letter], *Transfusion* 27: 503–4, 1987).

14. This is a complex issue. There are many reasons why some people in high-risk groups continue to serve as blood donors.

The worst cases, certainly, are those of people known to have AIDS or to be infected with the AIDS virus who repeatedly—and knowingly—continue to give blood. One such case, involving a man with AIDS who sold his infected blood to a Los Angeles commercial plasma bank, was reported recently ("Charges Filed Against Blood Donor in AIDS Case," *New York Times,* June 30, 1987, p. A18; *American Medical News,* July 24, 1987, p. 12). Similar cases are known to have occurred and are of grave concern, though it is hoped that they are very infrequent. Unfortunately, though, some individuals in high-risk groups continue to donate blood because of real or perceived social pressures (Consensus Conference, n. 3.26, p. 1782). In fact, this problem is probably of a much larger magnitude than has generally been acknowledged. Reporter Philip M. Boffey cited "several experts" who said that "many individuals in 'high risk' groups, such as male homosexuals, continue to donate blood despite all efforts to warn them away" (*New York Times,* July 8, 1986, p. C3). Some of the people at risk for HIV infection do not seem to realize that they might be infected—for example, a married man who has occasional sexual contact with other men may not consider himself bisexual. Others who certainly realize they might be infected donate blood as a way of proving to themselves that they are all right. There is also an unknown number of vengeful, bitter people who donate blood that they know may be infected, actually hoping that a contaminated unit slips through the testing maze and infects others.

15. This figure is based on data from the American Blood Commission cited by the CDC in *MMWR* 36: 137–40, 1987.

16. J. R. Bove, Transfusion-associated hepatitis and AIDS, *NEJM* 317: 242–45, 1987.

17. CDC, n. 5.2; Institute of Medicine/National Academy of Sciences, n. 1.3.

18. Klein and Alter, n. 2.28.

19. T. A. Peterman et al., Estimating the risks of transfusion-associated AIDS and HIV infection, *Transfusion* 27: 371, 1987.

20. Council on Scientific Affairs, Autologous blood transfusions, *JAMA* 256: 2378–80, 1986; M. S. Kruskall et al., Utilization and effectiveness of a hospital autologous preoperative blood donor program, *Transfusion* 26: 335–40, 1986; R. K. Haugen and G. E. Hill, A large-scale autologous blood program in a community

hospital, *JAMA* 257: 1211–14, 1987; D. R. Avoy, Autologous and aged blood donors [letter], *JAMA* 258: 1331, 1987. In addition, a Consensus Conference sponsored by the National Institutes of Health noted, "There is uniform agreement that autologous blood is the safest form of transfusion therapy" (*JAMA* 256: 1782, 1986).

21. P. T. Toy et al., Predeposited autologous blood for elective surgery, *NEJM* 316: 517–20, 1987.
22. D. M. Surgenor, The patient's blood is the safest blood, *NEJM* 316: 542–44, 1987.

CHAPTER 6

1. CDC, n. 2.38.
2. P. M. Boffey, "Failures Reported in AIDS Blood Tests," *New York Times,* July 8, 1986, p. C3.
3. "Organ Transplants Infect Two Patients Despite AIDS Tests," *New York Times,* May 29, 1987, p. A28.
4. A. W. Booth, AIDS and insects, *Science* 237: 355–56, 1987.
5. Ibid.
6. A letter to *Science* by D. F. Siemens, Jr. (AIDS transmission and insects, 238: 144, 1987), points out that if a mosquito, after having dined on an infected person, is squashed as it bites someone else, the blood from the mosquito's gut—which is splashed on the skin at the site of the bite—may contain enough viral particles to be infectious. If the person being bitten then scratches the itchy spot, "the standard method of transmission is present: virus-containing body fluid on a damaged epithelium."
7. M. W. Vogt et al., Isolation of HTLV-III from cervical secretions of women at risk for AIDS, *Lancet* 1: 525–27, 1986; Wofsy et al., n. 2.18; Archibald et al., n. 2.18.
8. D. Gianelli, "AIDS Protection Now Required," *American Medical News,* August 7, 1987, p. 1.
9. S. Fox, "HIV Risk in Office: Rectal, Colon Scopes," *Medical Tribune,* September 2, 1987, pp. 10–11.
10. CDC, Recommendations for preventing possible [transmission of] HTLV-III/LAV virus from tears, *MMWR* 34: 533–34, 1985. Similar precautions should be taken for other medical procedures, such as fitting women with diaphragms.

11. A. T. Ng et al., Tracing HIV-infected blood recipients: Large-scale recipient screening vs. look-back testing [letter], *JAMA* 258: 201–2, 1987.
12. F. Clavel et al., Isolation of a new human retrovirus from West African patients with AIDS, *Science* 233: 343–46, 1986; F. Clavel et al., Human immunodeficiency virus type 2 infection associated with AIDS in West Africa, *NEJM* 316: 1180–85, 1987.
13. L. K. Altman, "Third AIDS Virus Found in Sweden," *New York Times,* November 20, 1986, p. A24.
14. G. J. Stewart et al., Transmission of human T-cell lymphotropic virus type III by artificial insemination by donor, *Lancet* 2: 581–85, 1985; J. Morgan and J. Nolan, Risk of AIDS with artificial insemination, *NEJM* 314: 386, 1986; L. Mascola and M. Guinan, Screening to reduce transmission of sexually transmitted diseases in semen used for artificial insemination, *NEJM* 314: 1354–59, 1986.
15. CDC, n. 2.38.
16. Johnstone, n. 3.17.
17. L. K. Altman, "AIDS Virus: Always Fatal?" *New York Times,* September 8, 1987, p. C1.
18. J. L. Rhoads et al., Chronic vaginal candidiasis in women with human immunodeficiency virus infection, *JAMA* 257: 3105–7, 1987.
19. M. W. Vogt et al., Isolation patterns of the human immunodeficiency virus from cervical secretions during the menstrual cycle of women at risk for the acquired immunodeficiency syndrome, *Annals of Internal Medicine* 106: 380–82, 1987.
20. G. Y. Minuk, C. E. Bohme, and T. J. Bower, Condoms and hepatitis B virus infection, *Annals of Internal Medicine* 104: 584, 1986.
21. M. Conant et al., Condoms prevent transmission of AIDS-associated retrovirus, *JAMA* 255: 1706, 1986.
22. L. Resnick et al., Stability and inactivation of HTLV-III/LAV under clinical and laboratory environments, *JAMA* 255: 1887–91, 1986.
23. Ibid., p. 1890.
24. P. Boffey, "Worker Is Infected by AIDS Virus in Laboratory," *New York Times,* September 5, 1987, p. 6; P. Boffey, "Report on AIDS Lab Case," *New York Times,* September 12, 1987, p. 6; "2nd Worker Gets AIDS Virus," *New York Times,* October 10, 1987, p. 64.

25. According to Dr. Peter Fischinger, deputy director of the National Cancer Institute, the lab worker in question was infected "over a year ago [from the date it was publicly reported], but we didn't say anything because we hadn't isolated the virus" (D. M. Gianelli, "Researcher in AIDS Lab Infected with HIV," *American Medical News,* September 18, 1987, p. 2). Fischinger claimed that despite the fact that many lab workers came in contact with high concentrations of HIV, "there have been no other incidents." However, on October 8, 1987, the National Institutes of Health (which include the National Cancer Institute) announced the case of a second lab worker who was infected with HIV through occupational exposure in 1985, with the infection first detected in May 1986. An NIH spokesman claimed that because of a "communications breakdown," safety officials at NIH had only found out about the case recently (*New York Times,* October 10, 1987, p. 64).
26. J. H. Gilbaugh, Jr., and P. C. Fuchs, The gonococcus and the toilet seat, *NEJM* 301: 91–93, 1979.

CHAPTER 7

1. R. Lindsey, "AIDS Among Clergy Presents Challenges to Catholic Church," *New York Times,* February 2, 1987, p. A15.
2. A. C. Kinsey, W. B. Pomeroy, and C. E. Martin, *Sexual Behavior in the Human Male* (Philadelphia: Saunders, 1948); A. C. Kinsey et al., *Sexual Behavior in the Human Female* (Philadelphia: Saunders, 1953).
3. C. Tavris and S. Sadd, *The Redbook Report on Female Sexuality* (New York: Delacorte, 1977).
4. P. Blumstein and P. Schwartz, *American Couples* (New York: William Morrow, 1983); quoted material appears on pp. 270, 272.
5. "U.S. Syphilis Cases Rise 23%," *New York Times,* July 3, 1987, p. A15. As of October 31, 1987, there were 29,178 cases of syphilis reported in the U.S. for the year-to-date period, compared to 21,969 cases for the comparable period of 1986—a 33% increase (CDC, Table I—Summary: Cases of specified notifiable diseases, U.S., *MMWR* 36: 714, 1987).
6. Anyone who has spent much time working with gay men in the last few years realizes that a considerable number of these men altered their sex habits temporarily and then reverted to earlier

patterns of sexual behavior. This phenomenon, which the gay community does not like to discuss openly, is demonstrated in a recent study by Dr. Michael Quadland of Mount Sinai Medical School in New York City. Quadland used various techniques of sex education with a group of 619 gay and bisexual men to reduce risky sexual behavior. He found that gay and bisexual men who spent a weekend receiving education about safer sex practices (and discussing this information) generally had little change, with the exception of a group of men who watched erotic movies depicting safer sex practices. "Some men who received them [the safe sex guidelines] gave up sex completely for a time [of less than two months], but did not change their sexual behavior when they resumed having relations, Dr. Quadland said" (G. Kolata, "Erotic Films in AIDS Study Cut Risky Behavior," *New York Times,* November 3, 1987, p. C4).

7. M. Brading, "Doctors Assail Groups Billed As AIDS-Free," *Wall Street Journal,* September 30, 1987, p. 39.

8. CDC, HIV infection and pregnancies of sexual partners of HIV-seropositive hemophilic men—United States, *MMWR* 36: 593–95, 1987.

9. Conant et al., n. 6.21.

10. M. Conant, D.W. Spicer, and C. Smith, Herpes simplex virus transmission: Condom studies, *Sexually Transmitted Diseases* 11: 94–95, 1984.

11. Minuk, Bohme, and Bowen, n. 6.20; G. Y. Minuk et al., Condoms and the prevention of AIDS [letter], *JAMA* 256: 1443, 1986. See also mention of an unpublished study by Marcus Conant and his colleagues at the University of California at San Francisco indicating that "there was occasional leakage" of virus through natural membrane condoms (M. F. Goldsmith, Sex in the age of AIDS calls for common sense and condom sense, *JAMA* 257: 2261–66, 1987).

12. "FDA: One in Five Sample Lots of Condoms Failed Standards," *American Medical News,* September 4, 1987, p. 37.

13. L. Gruson, "Condoms: Experts Fear False Sense of Security," *New York Times,* August 18, 1987, p. C1.

14. J. D. Sherris, D. Lewison, and G. Fox, Update on condoms— products, protection, promotion, *Population Reports,* series H, no. 6, 1982; R. A. Hatcher et al., *Contraceptive Technology 1986–87* (New York: Irvington Publishers, 1986).

15. Padian et al., n. 2.11.
16. Goedert, n. 2.11.
17. To the best of our knowledge, there has not yet been any research showing that preejaculatory fluid contains HIV, but we believe it is prudent to assume for now that it probably does.
18. D. R. Hicks et al., Inactivation of HTLV-III/LAV-infected cultures of normal human lymphocytes by nonoxynol-9 in vitro, *Lancet* 1: 1422–23, 1985. In addition, Goldsmith (n. 7.11, p. 2263) reported on a recent study in which condoms permeated with nonoxynol-9 were deliberately torn; HIV was killed in two-thirds of these cases.
19. Winkelstein et al., n. 2.21.
20. Fischl et al., n. 2.14.

CHAPTER 8

1. CDC, Declining rates of rectal and pharyngeal gonorrhea among males—New York City, *MMWR* 33: 295–97, 1984.
2. L. McKusick et al., Reported changes in the sexual behavior of men at risk for AIDS, San Francisco, 1982–1984: The AIDS behavioral research project, *Public Health Reports* 100: 622–28, 1985; D. E. Reisenberg, AIDS-prompted behavior changes reported, *JAMA* 255: 171, 1986; S. Staver, "San Francisco Successful in Cutting HIV Infection Rate," *American Medical News,* November 27, 1987, p. 1.
3. Goedert, n. 2.11.
4. Winkelstein et al., n. 2.21.
5. This research was conducted by Robert C. Kolodny, M.D., through the Behavioral Medicine Institute, New Canaan, Connecticut.
6. This sad fact has been brought home to us in various research interviews over the last several years. It is also chronicled in Shilts, n. 3.27.
7. W. H. Masters, V. E. Johnson, and R. C. Kolodny, *Human Sexuality,* 3d ed. (Boston: Little, Brown, 1988), p. 437.
8. A. M. Rosenthal, "AIDS and Self-Interest," *New York Times,* September 22, 1987, p. A35.
9. J. Gross, "Bleak Lives: Women Carrying AIDS," *New York Times,* August 27, 1987, p. A1.
10. Chamberland and Dondero, n. 2.13, p. 764.

11. W. E. Schmidt, "High AIDS Rate Spurring Efforts for Minorities," *New York Times,* August 2, 1987, p. 1; G. Kolata, "Experts Say Women at Risk Are Well-Informed on AIDS," *New York Times,* September 30, 1987, p. A18.
12. M. Chase, "A Maverick, Bleak Numbers and Buses: Notes on International AIDS Conference," *Wall Street Journal,* June 6, 1987, p. 33.
13. Masters, Johnson, and Kolodny, n. 8.7.
14. R. C. Kolodny, W. H. Masters, and V. E. Johnson, *Textbook of Sexual Medicine* (Boston: Little, Brown, 1979).
15. M. Zelnik and J. F. Kantner, Sexual activity, contraceptive use, and pregnancy among metropolitan-area teenagers: 1971–1979, *Family Planning Perspectives* 12: 230–37, 1980; M. Zelnik, J. F. Kantner, and K. Ford, *Sex and Pregnancy in Adolescence* (Beverly Hills: Sage Publications, 1981); M. Zelnik and F. K. Shah, First intercourse among young Americans, *Family Planning Perspectives* 15: 64–70, 1983.
16. Alan Guttmacher Institute, *Teenage Pregnancy: The Problem That Hasn't Gone Away* (New York: Alan Guttmacher Institute, 1981); Zelnik, Kantner, and Ford, n. 8.15; E. A. McGee, *Too Little, Too Late: Services for Teenage Parents* (New York: Ford Foundation, 1982).
17. C. Chilman, *Adolescent Sexuality in a Changing American Society* (Bethesda: U.S. Department of Health, Education, and Welfare, #NIH 79-1426, 1979); Masters, Johnson, and Kolodny, n. 8.7.
18. S. Hofferth, J. R. Kahn, and W. Baldwin, Premarital sexual activity among U.S. teenage women over the past three decades, *Family Planning Perspectives* 19: 46–53, 1987.
19. L. D. Johnston, P. M. O'Malley, and Y. Bachman, *Drug Use Among American High School Students, College Students, and Other Young Adults: National Trends Through 1985* (Bethesda: U.S. Department of Health and Human Services, #ADM 86-1450, 1986); T. N. Robinson et al., Perspectives on adolescent substance use, *JAMA* 258: 2072–76, 1987.
20. Johnston, O'Malley, and Bachman, n. 8.19. According to data reported by the CDC, a 1986 survey of 15,200 high school seniors found that 12.7% had used cocaine in the last twelve months, 0.5% had used heroin, and 5.2% had used other opiates (CDC, Table 1—Trends in annual prevalence of drug use among high school seniors, *MMWR* 36: 721, 1987).

21. Data from Center for Population Options, Washington, D.C., cited in "Survey Shows Teenagers Misinformed About AIDS Transmission," *American Medical News,* June 5, 1987, p. 39.
22. Guttmacher Institute, n. 8.16.
23. Holmes et al., n. 1.5.
24. Zelnik and Kantner, n. 8.15.
25. D. Byrne and W. A. Fisher, *Adolescents, Sex, and Contraception* (Hillsdale, N.J.: Lawrence Erlbaum Associates, 1983).
26. "Survey Shows Teenagers Misinformed," n. 8.21.
27. S. L. Caron, R. M. Bertran, and T. McMullen, AIDS and the college student: The need for education, *SIECUS Report* 15 (6): 6–7, July–August 1987.
28. L. A. Kirkendall, *Premarital Intercourse and Interpersonal Relations* (New York: Julian Press, 1961); I. L. Reiss, *The Social Context of Premarital Sexual Permissiveness* (New York: Holt, Rinehart, & Winston, 1967); J. DeLamater and P. MacCorquodale, *Premarital Sexuality: Attitudes, Relationships, Behavior* (Madison: University of Wisconsin Press, 1979); I. L. Reiss, *Family Systems in America,* 3d ed. (New York: Holt, Rinehart, & Winston, 1980); I. L. Reiss, "Human Sexuality in Sociological Perspective," in Holmes et al., n. 1.5.

CHAPTER 9

1. Institute of Medicine/National Academy of Sciences, n. 1.3, p. 97.
2. Unlike some sex educators, we see no purpose to introducing AIDS education into the kindergarten or first-grade curriculum. Children at age 5 or 6 are too young to grasp what AIDS is and how it is transmitted. Furthermore, it is disturbing to think that young children will be taught that sex can kill before they fully understand that sex can be a source of joy and a form of deep intimacy. We feel that by age 10, most children have a better capacity to grasp this point.
3. Institute of Medicine/National Academy of Sciences, n. 1.3.
4. Ibid.
5. D. C. Bross, "Legal Aspects of STD Control," in Holmes et al., n. 1.5, pp. 925–30.
6. *New York Times,* April 23, 1987, p. A21.

7. T. Beardsley, U.S. troops and AIDS, *Nature* 316: 668, 1985.
8. L. Gostin, "Traditional Public Health Strategies," in H. L. Dalton, S. Burris, and the Yale AIDS Law Project, eds., *AIDS and the Law* (New Haven: Yale University Press, 1987), p. 57.
9. The quoted material is from Bross, n. 9.5; the lawsuit was Molien v. Kaiser Foundation Hospitals, August 25, 1980, California Supreme Court (*Family Law Reporter* 6: 2866–67, 1980).
10. D. P. Francis and J. C. Petricciani, The prospects for and pathways toward a vaccine for AIDS, *NEJM* 313: 1586–90, 1985; Institute of Medicine/National Academy of Sciences, n. 1.3; T. J. Matthews et al., Prospects for development of a vaccine against HTLV-III-related disorders, *AIDS Research and Human Retroviruses* 3 (supplement 1): 197–206, 1987; "Former FDA Head Cautions Against AIDS Vaccine Hopes," *American Medical News,* November 13, 1987.
11. The false positive rate of 1 in 10,000 for persons tested by ELISA confirmed by Western blot can be calculated from the parameters of the tests involved. A reasonable set of assumptions of the sensitivity and specificity of these tests is presented in an article by P. Cleary and his co-workers (*JAMA* 258: 1757–62, 1987), which we will discuss in detail later in this chapter. These workers calculated that a false positive rate of 1 in 10,000 would apply to a large-scale screening program involving a low-risk population. These types of calculations are strictly hypothetical, however. Thus, it is interesting to note that in the U.S. military testing program, a false positive rate of 1 in 135,000 has been achieved by virtue of stringent laboratory quality controls (Barnes, n. 5.9). That such a result is attainable outside the military can be seen in data from Minnesota, where the State Department of Health tested more than 250,000 low-risk persons without a single false positive result (C. SerVaas, "The News on AIDS Testing from Minnesota," *New York Times,* December 14, 1987, p. A22).
12. J. Gross, "Bathhouses and the AIDS Epidemic," *New York Times,* October 14, 1985, p. B3; S. Bronstein, "4 New York Bathhouses Still Operate Under City's Program of Inspections," *New York Times,* May 3, 1987. It should also be noted that various public health regulations have been used to close specific bathhouses that seemed especially flagrant in allowing high-risk sex on their premises, although such legal actions have not always been suc-

cessful. See, for example, G. W. Matthews and V. S. Neslund, The initial impact of AIDS on public health law in the United States—1986, *JAMA* 257: 344–52, 1987.

13. Dennis Altman discusses this matter in some detail in *The Homosexualization of America* (Boston: Beacon Press, 1983). He notes, "Large-scale luxurious pleasure palaces where everyone is potentially an immediate sexual partner are a common sexual fantasy; only for gay men are they a commonplace reality" (p. 17). "Men in bathhouses rarely talk much, and it is quite common for sex to take place without words, let alone names, being exchanged. . . . The willingness to have sex immediately, promiscuously, with people about whom one knows nothing and from whom one demands only physical contact, can be seen as a sort of Whitmanesque democracy" (p. 79).

14. Randy Shilts writes extensively in his book, *And the Band Played On* (n. 3.27), about the struggle to keep the gay bathhouses in San Francisco and New York open despite rising concerns that they were a breeding ground for AIDS. In one portion of this coverage, Shilts describes a meeting at the AIDS Clinic at San Francisco General Hospital, during which Dr. Paul Volberding, one of the nation's leading experts on AIDS, tried to convince bathhouse owners to close their establishments. "After Abrams [the assistant clinic director] and Volberding spoke, one of the owners of the largest bathhouses took them aside and tried to reason with them. 'We're both in it for the same thing,' he said. 'Money. We make money at one end when they come to the baths. You make money from them on the other when they come here.' Paul Volberding was speechless. This guy wasn't talking civil liberties; he was talking greed. Volberding felt helplessly naive. The bathhouses weren't open because the owners didn't understand they were spreading death. They understood that. The bathhouses were open because they were still making money" (pp. 421–22).

15. Chase, n. 8.12.

16. W. W. Darrow, "Prostitution and Sexually Transmitted Diseases," in Holmes et al., n. 1.5, pp. 109–16; J. W. Curran, "Prevention of Sexually Transmitted Diseases," in ibid., pp. 973–91.

17. Institute of Medicine/National Academy of Sciences, n. 1.3.

18. Padian, n. 2.13. See also a report of a study from Johns Hopkins

University discussed in *American Medical News* (October 23–30, 1987, p. 40) that found that 3% of females and 6.3% of males visiting a sexually transmitted disease clinic were infected with HIV, and that of these, one-third of the men and one-half of the women had become infected by heterosexual contact.

19. Guinan and Hardy, n. 4.5.
20. Scott et al.; Ledger; Mok et al., n. 2.34.
21. C. Marwick, HIV antibody prevalence data derived from study of Massachusetts infants, *JAMA* 258: 171–72, 1987.
22. A. M. Kaunitz et al., Prenatal care and HIV screening [letter], *JAMA* 258: 2693, 1987.
23. S. Landesman et al., Serosurvey of human immunodeficiency virus infection in parturients, *JAMA* 258: 2701–3, 1987.
24. Gross, n. 8.9; Schmidt, n. 8.11.
25. Baker et al., n. 2.39; J. L. Lennox, R. R. Redfield, and D. S. Burke, HIV antibody screening in a general hospital population, *JAMA* 257: 2914, 1987; H. H. Handesfield et al., Prevalence of antibody to human immunodeficiency virus and hepatitis B surface antigen in blood samples submitted to a hospital laboratory, *JAMA* 258: 3395–97, 1987. In the paper by Handesfield and co-workers, 3% of routine blood samples submitted to an urban teaching hospital's clinical chemistry laboratory were HIV-seropositive. The study was done in Seattle, which is not known as a particularly high-risk area for AIDS. Intriguingly, the 3% prevalence rate exactly matched the rate found by Baker and co-workers in their study (of a group of emergency room patients at Johns Hopkins in Baltimore).
26. R. R. Redfield et al., Disseminated vaccinia in a military recruit with human immunodeficiency virus (HIV) disease, *NEJM* 316: 673–76, 1987; CDC, Immunization of children infected with human T-lymphotropic virus type III/lymphadenopathy-associated virus, *Annals of Internal Medicine* 106: 75–78, 1987; D. R. Johns, M. Tierney, and D. Felenstein, Alteration in the natural history of neurosyphilis by concurrent infection with the human immunodeficiency virus, *NEJM* 316: 1569–72, 1987; C. D. Berry et al., Neurologic relapse after benzathine penicillin therapy for secondary syphilis in a patient with HIV infection, *NEJM* 316: 1587–89, 1987. In addition, physicians would want to know if their patients are infected with HIV before beginning any type

of treatment that might suppress immune functioning (e.g., corticosteroids, cancer chemotherapy).

27. CDC, n. 2.38.
28. J. B. Lucas, The national venereal disease problem, *Medical Clinics of North America* 56 (5): 1073–86, 1972.
29. Ibid.
30. Chase, n. 8.12; CDC, Heterosexual transmission of human T-lymphotropic virus type III/lymphadenopathy-associated virus, *MMWR* 34: 561–63, 1985; G. Papaevangelou et al., LAV/HTLV-III infection in female prostitutes [letter], *Lancet* 2: 1018, 1985; Kreiss et al., n. 1.9; M. Fischl et al., Human immunodeficiency virus (HIV) among female prostitutes in south Florida, in *Third International Conference*, n. 3.5.
31. P. D. Cleary et al., Compulsory premarital screening for the human immunodeficiency virus, *JAMA* 258: 1757–62, 1987.
32. Ibid., p. 1758.
33. A. S. Berenson, ed., *Control of Communicable Diseases in Man* (Washington, D.C.: American Public Health Association, 1985), p. 172.
34. Marwick, n. 9.21; Schoenbaum and Alderman, n. 4.5; Landesman et al., n. 9.23; Kaunitz et al., n. 9.22.
35. S. J. Ventura, Trends in marital status of mothers at conception and birth of first child, *NCHS Monthly Vital Statistics Report* 36 (2, supplement), 1987.
36. D. S. Burke, et al., Human immunodeficiency virus infections among civilian applicants for United States military service, October 1985 to March 1986, *NEJM* 317: 131–36, 1987; CDC, Trends in human immunodeficiency virus infection among civilian applicants for military service—United States, October 1985–December 1986, *MMWR* 36: 273–76, 1987; "Pentagon Testing Finds 3,035 in Military with AIDS Virus," *New York Times*, September 2, 1987, p. B4.
37. A. P. Bell and M. S. Weinberg, *Homosexualities* (New York: Simon & Schuster, 1978).
38. M. Saghir and E. Robins, *Male and Female Homosexuality* (Baltimore: Williams & Wilkins, 1973); L. Humphreys, *Tearoom Trade: Impersonal Sex in Public Restrooms* (Chicago: Aldine, 1970); E. Coleman, Bisexual and gay men in heterosexual marriage, *Journal of Homosexuality* 7: 93–103, 1982.
39. Marwick, n. 9.21.

40. Gross, n. 8.9. This estimate is at least partly supported by a survey that found an HIV antibody prevalence rate of 2.6% among 353 women seeking abortions in New York City (Schoenbaum and Alderman, n. 4.5).
41. D. M. Gianelli, "AIDS Testing Issues Divide Hearing Witnesses," *American Medical News,* August 21, 1987, p. 2.
42. Bross, n. 9.5; Dalton, Burris, and the Yale AIDS Law Project, n. 9.8.
43. Cleary et al., n. 9.31.
44. Institute of Medicine/National Academy of Sciences, n. 1.3; Peterman and Curran, n. 1.12.
45. H. Ennes and T. G. Bennett, The contact-education interview: Its functions, principles, and techniques in venereal disease contact investigation, *American Journal of Syphilis, Gonorrhea, and Venereal Disease* 29: 647, 1945.
46. Institute of Medicine/National Academy of Sciences, n. 1.3.
47. There is a good discussion of this extremely complex area of the law in R. Belitsky and R. Solomon, "Doctors and Patients: Responsibilities in a Confidential Relationship," in Dalton, Burris, and the Yale AIDS Law Project, n. 9.8, pp. 201–9. Despite the general conclusion in this chapter that a physician probably does have a legal duty to warn known sex partners of HIV-infected persons (at least if there is reason to believe they are not following "safer" sex guidelines), most physicians would probably shy away from this duty because they have been trained to treat confidentiality as an almost holy virtue. In fact, the Hippocratic Oath specifically defines it as such: "Whatsoever I shall see or hear in the course of my profession . . . if it be what should not be published abroad, I will not disclose it, holding such things to be holy secrets."
48. *New York Times,* October 14, 1987, p. B8.
49. In Nuremberg, a Bavarian court sentenced a former U.S. Army cook with AIDS to two years in prison for engaging in unprotected sex (S. Schmemann, "Bavarian Court Convicts American in AIDS Case," *New York Times,* November 17, 1987, p. A5). Similarly, an army sergeant (ironically, a medical instructor) was sentenced to five months in military prison and a dishonorable discharge in a plea bargaining agreement after admitting to having unprotected sex with three female soldiers despite knowing

he was HIV-positive and despite having been ordered by an officer either to tell his sexual partners he was seropositive or to wear a condom during sex ("Soldier with AIDS Virus to Be Imprisoned for Sexual Contacts," *New York Times,* December 4, 1987, p. B5).

INDEX

abstinence, 95–98, 127; among
homosexual men, 97–98; among
teenagers, 137, 138; during
testing for safe sex, 102–3;
among women vs. men, 96
acquired immune deficiency
syndrome. *See* AIDS
adolescents. *See* teenagers
Africa, 4, 17, 118; AIDS virus
strains in, 16, 88; heterosexual
transmission of AIDS in, 6;
number of AIDS cases in, 12, 14;
parasitic and microbial diseases
in, 37
AIDS (acquired immune deficiency
syndrome): clinical features of,
14, 17, 179–84; cure for, 153;
deaths from, 15; delayed
reporting of cases of, 13;
diagnosing of, 13, 14; estimates
of future trends in, 15; fear of, 2,
128–29, 136 as global epidemic,
11–15; misinformation about,
1–7; origin of, 16–17; prevention
of—*see* prevention of AIDS;
research on, 2, 148–49;
symptoms of, 35–40, 179–84;
underreporting of cases of,
12–14; vaccine for, 88, 153. *See
also* HIV

AIDS-related complex (ARC), 39,
40
AIDS virus. *See* HIV
Alter, M. J., 48–49
American Blood Commission, 76
American Hospital Association, 159
American Medical Association
(AMA), 77, 110, 146
American Medical News, 85
American Red Cross, 69, 71
American Society for
Gastrointestinal Endoscopy, 86
anabolic steroids, 26–27
anal intercourse, 6, 103, 130, 154;
condoms for, 118, 124, 126; HIV
transmission in, 21, 22, 23, 25;
among heterosexuals, 9–10,
59–60, 62, 63; among
homosexual men, 124, 125–26;
minimizing risks of, 118; study
findings on, 9–10, 59–60, 62, 63
anonymous sex: contact tracing
and, 173; among homosexual
men, 126–27, 154, 173;
antibodies, 41–42, 71, 74
antibody screening tests. *See*
ELISA; HIV antibody screening;
Western blot test
ARC (AIDS-related complex), 39,
40

ABOUT THE AUTHORS

WILLIAM H. MASTERS, M.D., Co-chairman of the Board of the Masters & Johnson Institute, is one of the pioneer sex researchers and therapists of the twentieth century. He is the author of more than 200 scientific publications, and the recipient of more than a dozen awards from professional organizations and universities. Among his many other activities, Dr. Masters currently serves as honorary Chairman of the AIDS Taskforce of the Society for the Scientific Study of Sex.

VIRGINIA E. JOHNSON, D.SC. (HON.), Co-chairman of the Board and Director of the Masters & Johnson Institute, is world-renowned for her innovative contributions to sex therapy and research. Co-author of 10 books and more than 200 journal articles, she is the holder of two honorary degrees and a wide range of professional awards in recognition of her achievements. Dr. Johnson's current research interests include women's studies and the psychobiology of sexual behavior.

ROBERT C. KOLODNY, M.D., is Medical Director and Chairman of the Board of the Behavioral Medicine Institute in New Canaan, Connecticut. Formerly Associate Director and Director of Training at the Masters & Johnson Institute, he continues to serve on its Board of Directors. In 1983 he received the National Award of the Society for the Scientific Study of Sex. Dr. Kolodny's publications include six books co-authored with Masters and Johnson.